T5-ASM-371

The People's Herbal

Other Books by Michael A. Weiner

Earth Medicine, Earth Foods
Plant a Tree
Man's Useful Plants
Homeopathy
In Search of the Durian
Ethnomedicine in Fiji
Weiner's Herbal
The Skeptical Nutritionist
The Art of Feeding Children Well

The People's Herbal

A Family Guide to
Herbal Home Remedies

DR. MICHAEL A. WEINER

A GD / Perigee Book

Perigee books
are published by
The Putnam Publishing Group
200 Madison Avenue
New York, New York 10016

Copyright © 1984 by Michael A. Weiner.
All rights reserved. This book, or parts thereof, may not be repro-
duced in any form without permission. Published simultaneously in
Canada by General Publishing Co. Limited, Toronto.

Library of Congress Cataloging in Publication Data

Weiner, Michael A.
    The people's herbal.

    Bibliography: p.
    Includes index.
    1. Herbs—Therapeutic use. 2. Medicine—
Formulae, receipts, prescriptions. 3. Therapeutics
—Popular works. 4. Folk medicine. I. Title.
RM666.H33W43 1984   615'.321   82-19062
ISBN 0-399-50772-8
ISBN 0-399-50756-6 (pbk.)

First Perigee printing, 1984
Printed in the United States of America.

1 2 3 4 5 6 7 8 9

The purpose of this book is to provide an interesting and historical document to the general public concerning herbal remedies that have been used for centuries. In presenting this information, we neither suggest or recommend its use. Nor is this volume intended as a substitute for personal medical care. *Only a physician familiar with herbal medicine may prescribe the use of these remedies, and he or she should be consulted as to which remedies, and in what dosage, should be used.*

Contents

8

Introduction

The Medicine Shelf

Your spice shelf probably contains several herbs with active medicinal properties. Thyme, for example, though used primarily for its savory flavor, has also been valued as a medicinal since ancient times. The leaves of this small, branched shrub contain the oil thymol, which has antiseptic, expectorant, and bronchodilator effects. Thymol also releases gas trapped in the stomach and relaxes the smooth muscle of this organ. This is why thyme is so effective in cases of colic and flatulence.

Ginger, another common spice, also has important medicinal values. As a tea, this widely used condiment is a popular remedy for encouraging menstruation when it has been suppressed by a cold. For headache and toothache, an infusion is rubbed directly on the affected part; the borneol in ginger relieves pain.

Garlic, now a staple for most cooks because of its unique flavor, contains selenium, an important trace mineral with remarkable biological effects. Long reputed for its ability to lower blood pressure, this tangy rhizome has antibacterial and diuretic properties as well. The juice is very effective for treating insect stings; and dripped into the ear (on a piece of cotton), it is a remarkable treatment for earaches!

Other common herbs with medicinal activity include pennyroyal, noted for stimulating the menses; peppermint, a truly effective gas expeller; dandelion, an ancient home remedy for mild constipation; anise, which increases milk secretion in nursing mothers; arrowroot (a valuable source of calcium), which was utilized by Central and South American Indians as an antidote for various poisons; and others.

Otto Mausert: Master Naturopath

The text on which this book is based comes to us from a naturopath who lived in the first half of this century, Otto Mausert. His book *Herbs for Health* was a record of nearly a half-century of successful healing with nature. Outdated information and recipes have been eliminated, while equivalent dosages, current Latin plant names,* and recent findings in pharmacology have been added. Many herbals contain single-plant remedies, but when it comes to complex mixtures or "recipes," Mausert's is interesting because it provides the effects of herbs in combination. In the recipes listed here, the most effective herbs are combined in the right proportions. In the sense that I am acting as a medical historian in rediscovering and updating Mausert's book, I make no claims about the healing properties of these remedies. They do, however, reflect how naturopathy was practiced over many centuries.

Naturopathy is a system of herbalism that employs no drugs and

---

*The Latin names given are those most commonly used in the herb trade today. Sources are E. Terrell, *A Checklist of Names for 3,000 Vascular Plants of Economic Importance,* USDA Agric. Handbook #505, Washington, D.C., 1977; J. Uphof, *Dictionary of Economic Plants* New York: J. Cramer, 1968; *J. Nickell's Botanical Ready Reference* Los Angeles: M. L. Baker, 1972; J. Remington and H. Wood, *Dispensatory of the United States of America,* (20th ed.), Philadelphia: Lippincott, (1918).

avoids chiropractic. Naturopaths are licensed to practice in many parts of the world and treat disease through the use of air, light, heat, nutrition, electrotherapy, physiotherapy, manipulations, minor surgery, and herbs. The discussions of "Symptoms and What They May Mean," pp. 21–26 and "Diseases, Their Symptoms, and Suggested Naturopathic Remedies," pp. 27–75 retain much of Mausert's original language, reflecting the theoretical orientation and attitude of the naturopath; where recent medical thinking provides an important added perspective, we have added the current knowledge of various disease states.

As the connections between botany and medicine become stronger, the value of Mausert's recipes will be recognized by the medical profession—a value already accepted by people who have been using them for over fifty years.

How to Gather, Prepare, and Preserve Herbs

Gathering Herbs. If you wish to collect your own herbs from the countryside or the herb garden, be sure to gather them at the peak of their growth, usually during the spring and early summer. The best time of day is in the early morning after the dew has dried; herbs that are moist when collected are not suitable for drying.

Leaves and flowers should be picked when young, just after opening. Discard discolored, withered, or insect-damaged plant parts, and snip off all stalks.

Seeds should be collected after sun-ripening on the plant.

Roots and barks should be gathered in the early spring, when the sap rises and the leaves are just budding, or after the plant has shed its leaves in the autumn.

Caution: Never collect any herbs that may have been contaminated with insecticides or other chemical sprays.

Drying Herbs. Herbs collected for drying must not be damp. Leaves and flowers should be hung in small bunches out of direct sun (except in cool climates) and where there is plenty of air circulation. They may also be spread on flat surfaces and turned frequently.

If you can, allow seeds to dry on the plant.

Handle fruits like leaves and flowers; larger fruits can be sun-dried in cooler climates, or they may be sliced, seeded, and dried slowly in an oven at low temperature with the door slightly open (turn them frequently).

Prepare roots and barks for drying by wiping them clean—do not wash them. In cold climates some artificial heat may be needed. They should be turned frequently during drying. They may also be cut up, strung with a needle, and hung in a well-ventilated room.

Storing Herbs. Dried herbs should be kept in a dry room that is not too hot. They can be stored in brown paper bags tied at the neck with a string, or they can broken up and stored in jars or tins.

Herbal Preparations. Medicinal plants can be eaten raw, and ideally this is the way to use them. But since many medicinal herbs have an unpleasant taste, and since they are often used dried, they are usually taken in the form of decoctions or infusions. Dried herbs are twice as strong as fresh, so when using fresh plant products larger amounts are necessary.

Decoctions are used for the tougher plant parts, such as roots and barks. They are made by boiling the vegetable material in water for a certain length of time, generally from 10 to 20 minutes, to extract the active or useful principles. Boil the mixture slowly in a covered vessel. Where proportions are not given, use about one teaspoon of the raw material to a cup of water.

Infusions are used for the softer plant parts—the leaves, flowers, and entire herbs. They are made in the manner of tea: Place the herb in a pot that has a tight cover. Pour boiling water over the vegetable material; then cover the pot and allow the infusion to stand until lukewarm. Strain and drink the infusion. Where the proportions are not given, use about one teaspoon of the raw material to a cup of water.

Introduction

Herbs as Prescription Drugs

We have noted that common kitchen spices often have strong medicinal properties. But did you know that you may already be getting herbal medicines in your prescriptions?

Over $3 billion is spent each year on pharmaceuticals derived from plants, not including microbes (which account for another $1.5 billion). To demonstrate the impact of plants as medicines, the twelve most commonly utilized pure compounds derived from drug plants and used in prescriptions are presented in Table 1.*

TABLE 1
Most Commonly Encountered Pure Compounds from Higher Plants Used as Drugs in 1973 in the U.S.A.

ACTIVE PLANT PRINCIPLE	TOTAL NUMBER OF PRESCRIPTIONS[a]	PERCENT OF TOTAL PRESCRIPTIONS
Steroids (95% from diosgenin)	225,050,000	14.69
Codeine	31,099,000	2.03
Atropine	22,980,000	1.50
Reserpine	22,214,000	1.45
Pseudoephedrine[b]	13,788,000	0.90
Ephedrine[b]	11,796,000	0.77
Hyoscyamine	11,490,000	0.75
Digoxin	11,184,000	0.73
Scopolamine	10,111,000	0.66
Digitoxin	5,056,000	0.33
Pilocarpine	3,983,000	0.26
Quinidine	2,758,000	0.18

[a]Total number of prescriptions in 1973 was 1.532 billion.
[b]These two are produced commercially by synthesis; all others by extraction from plants.

*Tables 1, 2, and 3 are from several papers written by Dr. Norman R. Farnsworth.

Introduction

Even more remarkable is the fact that over 38 million prescriptions written in 1973 contained crude plant drugs or extracts from plants. Those most commonly prescribed are listed in Table 2.

TABLE 2

Most Commonly Encountered Higher Plant
Extracts Used in Prescriptions in 1973

CRUDE BOTANICAL OR EXTRACT	TOTAL NUMBER OF PRESCRIPTIONS[a]	PERCENT OF TOTAL PRESCRIPTIONS
Belladonna *(Atropa belladonna)*	10,418,000	0.62%
Ipecac *(Cephaelis ipecacuanha)*	7,047,000	0.46%
Opium *(Papaver somniferum)*	6,894,000	0.45%
Rauwolfia *(Rauvolfia serpentina)*	5,822,000	0.38%
Cascara *(Rhamnus purshiana)*	2,451,000	0.16%
Digitalis *(Digitalis purpurea)*	2,451,000	0.16%
Citrus Bioflavonoids *(Citrus* spp.*)*	1,379,000	0.09%
Veratrum *(Veratrum viride)*	1,072,000	0.07%

[a]Total prescription volume in 1973 was 1.532 billion prescriptions.

Natural plant drugs have been used since antiquity, and are still the only form of medicine for a large majority of the world's population who do not have access to hospitals and pharmacies. Herbal medicine is often based on rational principles, as we see in Table 3. The left column contains the names of compounds derived from plants; in the middle column are the type of chemicals they contain; and on the right we see the type of effects they produce in the body.

So using herbal medicine is not so far removed from our daily lives as we may think. Many prescription drugs contain herbal compounds not unlike the remedies listed in *The People's Herbal.*

TABLE 3

Typical Plant Principles Used to Illustrate Pharmacological
Principles in Standard Textbooks

NAME OF COMPOUND	TYPE OF COMPOUND	TYPE OF PHARMACOLOGICAL ACTION
Bulbocapnine	Alkaloid	Centrally acting skeletal muscle relaxant
Morphine, Codeine	Alkaloid	Analgesic
Papaverine	Alkaloid	Smooth muscle relaxant
Colchicine	Alkaloid	Anti-gout
Camphor	Monoterpene	Stimulates central nervous system
Picrotoxin	Sesquiterpene	
Strychnine, Caffeine, Theobromine, Theophylline	Alkaloid	
Cocaine	Alkaloid	Local anesthetic
Atropine, Scopolamine	Alkaloid	Parasympatholytic
Pilocarpine, Physostigmine	Alkaloid	Parasympathomimetic
d-Tubocurarine	Alkaloid	Peripherally acting skeletal muscle relaxant
Ephedrine	Alkaloid	Sympathomimetic
Nicotine, Lobeline	Alkaloid	Ganglionic blocker
Digitoxin, Digoxin	Cardiac glycoside	Cardiotonic
Quinidine	Alkaloid	Antiarrhythmic
Sparteine, Ergot Alkaloids	Alkaloid	Uterine stimulant
Reserpine, *Veratrum* Alkaloids	Alkaloid	Antihypertensive
Reserpine	Alkaloid	Psychotropic
Anthraquinone glycosides	Anthraquinone	Cathartic
Psyllium, Agar	Mucilages	Laxative
Castor Oil	Fixed Oil	Laxative
Quinine	Alkaloid	Antimalarial
Emetine	Alkaloid	Antiamebic

The People's Herbal

1

Symptoms and What They May Mean

The following descriptions of symptoms are based on those provided by Otto Mausert, renowned naturopath, who had decades of experience in treating illness. We make no medical claims in this book, reprinting this manuscript for historical purposes only. In the case of pathological conditions, the reader is advised to consult a physician, and to incorporate Mausert's remedies into their treatment on the basis of a mutual decision between patient and doctor.

Pain in the Head (Headaches)

The underlying cause of this pain can often be found in stomach disorders, constipation, anemia, menstrual irregularities, high blood pressure, eye strain, or disturbances of lung or heart function.

Pain in the Back and Pelvis

Back pains are often observed in *articular rheumatism* (pain over the whole spinal column); *lumbago* (pain confined to the lumbar region); *kidney diseases* (pain in the middle or lower trunk, to the right or left of the spine); *gallstones or inflammation of the gallbladder* (pain extends from the lowest rib on the right side toward the right shoulder blade). *Pelvic pain* may indicate affections of the ovaries, fallopian tubes, or uterus; rectal diseases; or hemorrhoids.

Pain in the Chest

In *pleurisy* the pain is sharp and stinging, especially when taking a deep breath, with low-grade fever generally present. In *pneumonia* the pain is accompanied by dry, painful, hacking cough, high fever, and chills. In *neuralgia or rheumatism* pressure increases the pain; breathing is sometimes painful. In *shingles* there are severe neuralgic pains with small, bright red, blistery eruptions on the inflamed skin.

Pain in the Stomach

In *gastritis*, the pain is gnawing and burning at the pit of the stomach after eating (so-called heartburn), with gas present and a tenderness in the epigastric region. Vomiting may occur at times, but without giving relief from pain, and slight fever may be noticed. In *dyspepsia*, there is pain as in gastritis, but less severe, without fever or tenderness. Vomiting occurs occasionally, which gives relief from pain. In *gastric ulcer*, there is pain below the breastbone, very sensitive to pressure, often radiating backward toward the shoulder blade, and almost always encountered after eating. Vomiting of a sour fluid is common, and there is sometimes loss of blood; the stools are at times black and tarry, due to the passage of coagulated blood. It is important to seek medical attention to distinguish ulcer symptoms from those of stomach cancer. In *neuralgia or cramps in the stomach*, there are sudden attacks of severe gripping pains in the stomach, usually extending toward the back and lasting from a few minutes to sometimes several hours; the pain ceases suddenly with the expulsion of gas or a watery liquid, leaving the patient in a very exhausted condition.

Pain in the Abdomen

In *diarrhea,* with frequent watery and slimy stools. In *dysentery,* with the passage of mucus tinged with blood.

Pain in the Rectum

In *hemorrhoids or piles,* with itching or occasional passage of clear blood from the rectum. (Seek medical attention in the case of blood loss; it may indicate cancer.) In *catarrh or inflammation of the bowels,* with lumpy or stringy stools. In *dysentery,* with burning, coliclike pains and a discharge of bloody, slimy stools and pus. In *constipation,* due to the pressure used to force bowel movements.

Pain in the Bladder

In *catarrh of the bladder*: Spasmodic pains in the urinary bladder with frequent and painful urination. In *gravel or stone in the bladder*: Pain in the neck of the bladder extending along the urinary tract; flow of urine at times interrupted or stopped. In *displacement and falling of the uterus*: Dull bearing-down pains, with a constant desire to urinate when uterus rests on the bladder. In *gonorrhea*: Burning pain when urinating, sometimes accompanied by discharge of pus from the urinary canal, especially in men.

Pain in the Throat

In *tonsillitis*: Painful swallowing, with an inflamed condition of the mucous membrane of the throat and the roof of the mouth. In *diphtheria*: Pain with a dirty-white membrane covering the throat.

Vomiting

In *acute dyspepsia,* vomiting occurs shortly after eating; and in *chronic dyspepsia,* generally in the morning. In *ulcer of the stomach,* vomiting occurs immediately after meals; the vomitus at times contains or may consist entirely of blood. These symptoms may also indicate cancer; a physician should be consulted. In *dilation (swell-*

ing) of the stomach, vomiting occurs at long intervals, often of several days, and consists of large amounts of fermented food. Continuous vomiting may indicate cholera or a severe intestinal inflammation. In such diseases of children as scarlet fever, diphtheria, measles, and tonsillitis, vomiting is often one of the first and outstanding symptoms.

Vomiting also occurs in pregnancy, or with gallstones, kidney stones, uterine diseases, or intestinal colic. Vomiting of fecal matter indicates intestinal obstructions, twisted intestines, strangulation of a hernia.

Stools

Color: In diseases of the liver, jaundice, gallstones, and inflammation of the gallbladder, the stools are at times *clay-colored or whitish,* and sometimes *greenish* from bile. Medicines such as bismuth and iron may produce a *black-colored* stool. Black, tarry stools point to hemorrhages from stomach or bowels (ulcer or cancer). In intestinal catarrh of babies the stools are *greenish;* in diarrhea, *yellowish-brown;* and in cholera, *whitish-dirty.*

Blood in stools, clear and unchanged: Hemorrhoids or piles, rectal hemorrhages, typhoid fever, dysentery. *Blood in stools, coagulated, tarry-looking:* Ulcer or cancer of stomach or small intestine.

Pus in stools: Ulcer or cancer of the rectum, chronic dysentery, appendicitis.

Mucus in stools: Catarrh of stomach and bowels, diarrhea, inflammation of the bowels, or catarrh of the colon (colitis).

Dizziness (Vertigo)

May accompany disorders of the stomach, bowels, or liver; dyspepsia, constipation, obstruction of the hepatic ducts. In nervous disorders (nervous vertigo), with the so-called sick or nervous headache.

Itching of the Skin

May indicate diseases of the liver, gallstones, inflammation of the gallbladder, jaundice, blood poisoning; in advanced cases of kidney diseases and diabetes. In various forms of eczema, hives, barber's itch; bites of fleas, bedbugs, lice, crab lice, scabies.

Tired Feeling
Often due to self-poisoning of the system; constipation, sluggish liver function, anemia, heart diseases, obesity.

Sleeplessness
Nervous exhaustion; cough; asthma; overwork; abuse of alcohol, coffee, tea, or tobacco; fever, excitement, worries.

Cough
Inflammation and catarrhal conditions of the bronchial tubes and lungs. Pleurisy, pneumonia, laryngitis, tuberculosis, whooping cough, and the so-called stomach cough, due to irritation of the larynx by the belching of acids and gas from the stomach. Certain forms of nervousness and hysteria (nervous cough).

Shortness of Breath
In pleurisy, with stinging pain in the side. In pneumonia, with sharp pain near the nipple. Tuberculosis, heart diseases, chronic emphysema; different forms of dropsy due to the accumulation of water; pressure from gas in the stomach and abdomen. Obstructions from enlarged tonsils, adenoids, polyps in the nose. Diphtheria, catarrhal affections of the bronchial tubes and lungs, or asthma.

Ringing in the Ears
Diseases of the ear and especially in catarrhal or inflamed conditions of the middle ear and Eustachian tube (a tube leading from the roof of the mouth to the ear); cardiovascular diseases, including high blood pressure; tumors. Anemic and nervous people often complain about these noises, the latter especially about getting them at night while in bed. Obstructions by earwax and overuse of quinine or salicylate (aspirin) preparations are often responsible for this trouble.

Sweating

In anemic and obese people; in weakness of the heart or lungs, and in general weakness. Diseases associated with fever. Local excessive sweating is often a sign of nervous troubles. The secretion of a yellowish sweat indicates disorders of liver and gallbladder.

Coated Tongue

In catarrh of the stomach, the coating is grayish-white with a pasty taste and a foul breath, the tongue often showing the impression of the teeth. A dry, thick tongue with numerous cracks and enlarged, reddened papillae often indicates diabetes.

Swelling

Slight swelling of the ankles, disappearing during the night, often indicates an anemic condition. Extensive swelling, especially when extending upward to the knees and hips, is noticed in diseases of the heart, lungs, kidneys, liver, and in obstruction caused by tumors or other growths.

Color of Skin and Face

Pale: In anemia, as an aftereffect after hemorrhages of stomach, liver, bowels, kidneys, and bladder; fainting spells, seasickness, migraine.

Red: Fevers. In tuberculosis, a hectic redness of the cheeks. In menopause, red, hot flushes toward the head. Enlargement of the blood vessels, especially of the nose and cheeks. Inflammation, with the presence of heat.

Yellow: In catarrhal inflammation of the bile ducts or duodenum; diseases of liver and gallbladder; cancer. In anemic conditions, pale dirty-yellow.

2

Diseases, Their Symptoms, and Suggested Naturopathic Remedies

The herbal recipes referred to are to be found in the section beginning on page 82; for convenience in locating specific recipes, they are all listed on pages 76–79.)

Abscess
See IMPURE BLOOD; SORES, OPEN.

Acidity
See STOMACH DISORDERS.

Acne
See IMPURE BLOOD.

Diseases, Symptoms, and Suggested Remedies

Anemia

A deficiency of red blood cells, in quantity and/or quality.

Treatment: Sunshine, fresh air, rest, and a well-balanced diet, including a quantity of fresh green vegetables and the daily use of good tonics. (For a good herbal tonic, refer to No. 11.)

Appetite, Lack of

See STOMACH DISORDERS.

Arthritis

See RHEUMATISM.

Asthma

This disease manifests itself in temporary attacks of difficult breathing, usually with a sense of suffocation, a wheezing noise, and cough. It is generally due to an extreme irritability of the mucous membrane of the air passages. This affection is frequently associated with diseases of the nasal or bronchial mucous membrane, chronic heart disease, disturbances of the stomach and bowels, disturbances of the nervous system, a sensitivity to certain odors, pollen, dust, smoke, etc.

Treatment: The treatment should be general, constitutional, tonic, and eliminative. Special attention should be paid to the functions of stomach, liver, and bowels. The diet should be nonstimulating. Sweets and starches should be used with extreme moderation. Ripe fruits and vegetables should constitute the greater portion of the meal. Overloading, especially with rich food, should be avoided. Plenty of moderate outdoor exercise is beneficial. If constipated, bowels should be regulated by all means (see Constipation). Warm mustard compresses applied alternately to calves of the legs and the chest are also very beneficial.

Remedies: To relieve the paroxysms, use by inhalation either Inhalation Powder, No. 3, or Asthma Cigarettes, No. 4. Internally, use No. 2.

Assisting the Treatment: If constipated, use No. 26 or 27; if the liver is sluggish, then use No. 6 instead of No. 26 or 27.

If stomach is out of order, use No. 92 or 93; where a tonic is needed, use No. 11 in conjunction with the treatment.

Backache
See RHEUMATISM; KIDNEYS, INFLAMMATION OF.

Bad Breath
See STOMACH DISORDERS; CONSTIPATION.

Bed-wetting
This disagreeable trouble is due to an involuntary relaxation and weakness of the muscle that closes the bladder.
Remedy: Use No. 5.
Assisting the Treatment: In nervous weakness, use No. 66. In bodily weakness, use No. 11.

Belching
See STOMACH DISORDERS.

Biliousness (congestion of the liver; sluggish or torpid liver)
This complaint consists of a group of symptoms affecting stomach, liver, gallbladder, and bowels. Inflammation of the mucous membrane is generally present and brings on the attacks, which are popularly known as biliousness. This disorder is indicated by a feeling of fullness, heaviness, and pain over the region of the stomach, which continues until nausea, and often vomiting of a greenish or yellowish slimy matter, occurs. The appetite is poor, the tongue coated, the taste bitter and pasty. The urine is dark, amber-colored, and scanty. The bowels are usually constipated. The complexion is sallow with a yellowish tint, especially around the eyes. A dull aching pain in the head, sometimes rather severe and commonly known as "sick headache," is often present.
Treatment: As overeating, especially of too much greasy food, is often responsible for the attacks, a light, nonirritating diet should be

resorted to. The stomach, liver, and bowels should be properly regulated. (See also GALLBLADDER, INFLAMMATION OF.)

Remedy: Use No. 6.

Assisting the Treatment: If stomach is not working properly, use No. 90 or 92, in conjunction with No. 6. If the gallbladder is affected, use Nos. 47 and 48, in which case do not use No. 6.

Biting the Fingernails

This bad and unsightly habit should be corrected by all means. It not only looks bad, but often it is dangerous. Pieces of nails may be swallowed, which may cause dangerous irritations.

Remedy: Use No. 7.

Assisting the Treatment: To be used in conjunction with No. 7. If the condition is due to nervousness, use No. 66 or 67. If constipated, use No. 26 or 27 or 28.

Blackheads

See IMPURE BLOOD.

Bladder, Inflammation or Catarrh of (Cystitis)

This trouble is characterized by a constant desire to urinate. The urine is hot, cloudy, and thick, flowing only scantily, often only drop by drop, at times passing with pain, or sometimes stopping entirely. Slight fever with a dry, hot skin may be present. The bowels are, as a rule, constipated.

Treatment: Hot compresses, or, still better, hot sitz baths (see SITZ BATHS, HOT) should be given. Flax seed tea should be used freely instead of water. Ice cold drinks must be avoided.

Remedy: Use No. 8.

Assisting the Treatment: To be used in conjunction with No. 8: If constipated, use No. 26 or 27. In female complaints, use No. 60 or 62. If gravel or stones are present in the bladder, use No. 96 instead of No. 8.

Bladder, Gravel or Stones in

See STONES OR GRAVEL IN KIDNEYS OR BLADDER.

Bloating

See STOMACH DISORDERS.

Blood, Impure

See IMPURE BLOOD.

Blood Pressure, High (Hypertension)

Overindulgence in fatty foods, in alcoholic drinks, in tobacco, or overwork is often responsible for high blood pressure. These habits often lead to hardening of the arteries, a condition primarily responsible for the trouble. Other possible causes include nervous weakness, continuous excitement, kidney disease, menopause, toxic conditions, etc. Ringing noises in the ear can also often be traced to high blood pressure, being due to the overfilling of the blood vessels of the brain with blood.

Treatment: Rest and quiet. The diet should be light, low in salt, and of a nonstimulating nature. The bowels should be kept well regulated. Excitement should be avoided. Chronic high blood pressure should receive medical attention.

Remedies: Use No. 9 or 10.

Assisting the Treatment: To be used in conjunction with either No. 9 or 10, unless otherwise stated: In nervous weakness, use No. 66 or 67 or 68. In menopause, use No. 18. In indigestion, use No. 92. In kidney irregularities, use No. 57. In biliousness, use No. 6 instead of No. 10.

Blood Pressure, Low

In this condition, it is generally advisable to build up the system through a well-balanced diet, with a liberal quantity of fresh vegetables and ripe fruits when in season. The daily use of tonics is also very beneficial.

Remedy: Use No. 11.

Bloody Stools

See DYSENTERY.

Body Odor (Offensive perspiration)

Remedy: Deodorizing Lotion, No. 12.

Boils and Inflamed Pimples

These are generally due to an infection of the sweat glands or hair roots, or to the accumulation of impurities in the blood caused by some derangement of stomach, bowels, or liver.

Remedies: To help maturation of the boils, apply externally Nos. 13 and 103. As a depurative, or blood cleanser, use No. 54 or 55.

Assisting the Treatment: If the liver is sluggish and a stronger laxative is needed, use No. 6 instead of No. 54 or 55. If the stomach is out of order, use No. 90 or 91 in conjunction with Nos. 54 or 55 or 6.

Bowels, Inflammation of

See DIARRHEA.

Breath, Bad or Foul

See STOMACH DISORDERS.

Bronchitis (Bronchial catarrh)

An inflammation of the lining of the bronchial mucous membrane. The air passages feel dry, and coughing is generally painful; hoarseness and soreness are often noticed.

Remedy: Use No. 14 or 15.

Assisting the Treatment: To be used in conjunction with either No. 14 or 15, unless otherwise stated: In case of catarrh, use No. 64. If constipated, use No. 26 or 27 or 28.

For a cold, use No. 20, and in order to produce sweating, use before retiring No. 21 or 22. Since No. 20 also possesses laxative properties, other laxatives should not be used with it.

Bruises and Sprains

Remedy: Use liniment, No. 84.

Bunions

An inflamed and painful swelling of the lubricating sac of the joint of the great toe, generally due to pressure from tight shoes. If not relieved, disfigurement and enlargement of the joint may take place.

Remedy: External application of No. 16 or 17.

Assisting the Treatment: If inflamed, use No. 81 until inflammation is relieved and then treat as indicated above.

Burns

See WOUNDS.

Buzzing in the Ears

See EARACHE; BLOOD PRESSURE, HIGH.

Canker Sores

Remedy: External application of No. 98.

Calluses

See CORNS AND CALLUSES.

Carbuncles

See BOILS AND INFLAMED PIMPLES.

Catarrh

See NASAL CATARRH.

Catarrh of the Bladder

See BLADDER, INFLAMMATION OR CATARRH OF.

Catarrh of the Bowels

See DIARRHEA.

Catarrh of the Bronchial Tubes

See BRONCHITIS.

Catarrh of the Head
See COLD OR ACUTE CATARRH IN THE HEAD.

Catarrh of the Nose
See NASAL CATARRH.

Catarrh of the Stomach
See STOMACH DISORDERS.

Chafing
Remedy: Antiseptic Salve, No. 103.

Change of Life
See MENOPAUSE.

Chapped Skin or Chapped Hands, Face, or Lips
See WOUNDS.

Chilblains (Frostbite)
An inflammation of the skin produced by exposure to cold. The parts frequently affected are the ears, fingers, toes, and nose. A slight swelling with redness, tickling, itching, and smarting characterizes the trouble.

Remedies: External application of No. 19. If skin is broken, apply externally No. 17.

Chills
See COLD OR ACUTE CATARRH IN THE HEAD.

Circulation, Poor
See COLD FEET AND HANDS.

Coated Tongue
See STOMACH DISORDERS; BILIOUSNESS; "Symptoms," p. 26.

Coffee or Tea Substitute

See No. 71, and *Maté*, p. 212.

Cold or Acute Catarrh in the Head (Acute nasal catarrh)

This inflamed condition of the mucous membrane of the nose and throat often causes considerable trouble by obstructing the nasal passages with mucus. Headaches, chills, sneezing, running of the nose and eyes, loss of smell and taste, and impaired hearing may result. If neglected, this temporary indisposition may lead to more serious trouble; it should therefore be attended to promptly.

Treatment: The first thing to do in colds is to cause the proper elimination of morbid matter from the system. This is best accomplished by opening the bowels, and also the pores of the skin. Rest in bed is advisable in cases of extreme weakness or fever.

Remedies: To open bowels and lower fever use No. 30; if the cough is deep-seated, then use No. 15 instead of No. 30.

Cold Feet and Hands

Poor circulation, insufficient blood supply to affected parts, or disturbances in the digestive and nervous system are generally responsible for this trouble. In order to overcome this condition, it is first necessary to find the cause and treat it. To aid the parts affected, it is well to aid in stimulating the circulation by applying hot and cold wet compresses to them alternately. After thoroughly drying the surfaces, massage them well with a penetrating cream.

Remedy: For a penetrating cream, use No. 23.

Assisting the Treatment: To be used in connection with No. 23: In case of nervousness, use No. 66 or 67 or 68. In case of indigestion, use No. 90 or 92 or 93. In case of blood deficiency, use No. 11.

Cold Sores

See HEALING BALSAM; WOUNDS; STOMACH DISORDERS.

Colic, Bilious

See BILIOUSNESS.

Colic in Children

This common, troublesome disorder in infants is generally caused by cold food that disagrees, gas in stomach and bowels, constipation, worms, etc. The child is generally restless, draws up its legs, kicks, and screams. The urine may often flow scantily or stop temporarily. It is of the utmost importance to identify and correct the underlying condition causing the problem. A small enema with soap water, or still better a small enema with a mild infusion of chamomile flowers, followed by a gentle circular massage of the abdomen, beginning from the right to the left, will generally give quick relief.

Remedy: To aid the digestion and help to expel gases, use No. 24.

Assisting the Treatment: To be used in conjunction with No. 24: If constipated, use No. 28. If worms are present, use No. 102.

Colon Flush

See ENEMA.

Complexion, Pale and Sallow

See BILIOUSNESS; CONSTIPATION; STOMACH DISORDERS; "Symptoms," p. 26.

Color of Skin and Face

See "Symptoms," p. 26.

Constipation

Health depends greatly upon the regular and normal action of the bowels, because inactive bowels cause congestion of the entire digestive tract; food then taken into the system does not digest properly and becomes subject to decay. The products of decomposition are of a poisonous nature and, when absorbed into the system, tend to poison it and consequently lead to disease. Lack of appetite, headache, dizziness, coated tongue, bad breath, impure blood, pale complexion, and inactivity of the liver may result from this poisoning of the system, which if not relieved may lead to other, more serious diseases.

Since most cases of constipation are brought on by an incorrect and unnatural way of living, we must first of all correct our habits and restore them to harmony with the laws of nature. We must chew our food slowly and well and not overeat. Food not sufficiently masticated cannot be properly attacked by the digestive juices, and if not properly digested, turns sour and ferments. This produces excessive amounts of gas and acids and the food becomes subject to decay in the bowels. This condition in turn creates heat and dryness and causes the fecal matter to harden, thus hindering the normal evacuation of the bowels.

Very often the fermentation of the food begins in the stomach and the formation of gas causes the stomach to become enlarged. As the liver and gallbladder lie directly over the side of the stomach, this enlargement presses against them and interferes with the normal flow of the liver's secretion, which is known as bile and which acts as a lubricant for the bowels. As a result, the bowels become sluggish from the lack of the natural lubricant and normal evacuation of the bowels is hindered. It is therefore essential in the treatment of constipation to encourage and stimulate the normal flow of bile by acting on the liver, the organ that produces it.

Attend promptly to the call of nature and assist the function of the bowels by a natural way of living. Their activity should be encouraged and not interfered with. Where a temporary condition of constipation exists, attend to it promptly; otherwise a chronic condition may set in.

Remedies: At the first sign of constipation, use No. 25, which should be made into capsules. This excellent recipe acts on the liver and aids the flow of bile. Nos. 26 and 27 are also very helpful in the treatment of constipation. For children, use No. 28.

Assisting the Treatment: (1) Regular attendance to the call of nature. (2) Changing the diet to a more eliminative one, by eating more green vegetables, salads, fruits, and other foods that give bulk to the intestines. (3) Occasional enemas, once or twice a month.

Corns and Calluses

A thickening of the skin caused by pressure or friction.

Remedy: No. 29, applied externally to the affected area.

Diseases, Symptoms, and Suggested Remedies

Cough

An inflamed condition of the air passages, brought about by colds and irritation of the mucous lining. (See also WHOOPING COUGH; "Symptoms." p. 25.)

Remedies: A good expectorant tea is No. 30. In coughs of long standing, use No. 14 or 15, instead of No. 30. (See also BRONCHITIS.)

Assisting the Treatment: If complicated with a cold, use No. 20.

Cramps in Bowels

See DIARRHEA.

Cramps in Female Organs

See MENSTRUATION.

Cramps in Stomach

See STOMACH DISORDERS.

Cuts

See HEALING BALSAM; WOUNDS.

Cystitis

See BLADDER, INFLAMMATION OR CATARRH OF.

Dandruff

A disorder due to faulty function of the sebaceous glands of the scalp, characterized by the casting off of whitish-gray scales and the falling out of the hair. A disturbed condition of the system in general is often a contributing cause of this trouble, and should, therefore, be considered in the treatment.

Remedies: Use as a shampoo twice a week No. 31, and apply daily to the scalp No. 32.

Assisting the Treatment: To be used in conjunction with the above: In nervous condition, use No. 66 or 67 or 68. If indigestion is present, use No. 92 or 93. If constipated, use No. 6 or 26 or 27.

Diabetes

The origin of this disease can be traced back to derangement of the functions of the pancreas gland. Contributing factors, however, may undoubtedly include severe nervous disturbances, and improper functions of stomach, liver, and bowels. The patient feels tired and weak, usually complains about pains in the limbs, feeling depressed and downhearted. An abnormal thirst is often experienced. Dizziness and headaches are common. The skin is dry and often itchy. The digestion is often upset, due to the abnormal increased appetite. The eyesight may be impaired and weak. The urine is generally very pale and plentiful. An excessive amount of sugar is present in the urine.

For the continuous thirst, flax seed tea, with a small quantity of peppermint herb, may be used freely. The diet should be carefully watched. Sugars and refined starches should be eliminated. Pure gluten bread should be eaten instead of ordinary bread. Soy flour may be used instead of ordinary flour. The bowels should be kept well regulated. Rest and sunshine are beneficial.

Remedy: Use No. 33.

Assisting the Treatment: To be used in conjunction with No. 33: If the liver is sluggish, use No. 6 or 47. If constipated, use No. 25 or 26 or 27, instead of No. 6 or 47. If stomach is out of order, use No. 92 or 93. In nervous disturbances, use No. 66 or 67 or 68.

Diaphoretic Tea

See Nos. 21 and 22.

Diarrhea (Catarrh or inflammation of the bowels; looseness of the bowels)

Usually caused by exposure to cold or extreme heat, indigestion, irritating or spoiled food, ice cold drinks, unripe fruit, mental disturbances. Hot sitz baths (see SITZ BATHS, HOT) or the application of heat to abdomen is very helpful. (See also DYSENTERY.)

Remedies: The following remedies will be found very beneficial. No. 34; in more severe cases No. 35 should be taken in conjunction with No. 34.

Assisting the Treatment: To be taken in conjunction with the above: If stomach is disordered, use No. 90 or 91 or 92. In nervousness, use No. 66 or 67 or 68.

Dizziness

See CONSTIPATION; BILIOUSNESS; STOMACH DISORDERS; BLOOD PRESSURE, HIGH.

Dropsy (Edema).

This, in itself, is not a disease. It is the result of a change in the blood by obstructions to the blood flow. It may be the result of poor or faulty function of the inner vital organs, especially the heart, lungs, or kidneys. It is important that the cause be treated. To help relieve the dropsical condition, the activity of the urinary organs, the skin, and the bowels should be increased.

For the bowels, hydragogues should be used. The kidneys should be helped to increase the elimination of urine. The pores of the skin should also be opened.

Remedies: Use No. 36 or 37 in conjunction with No. 38. To induce sweating, use No. 21 or 22.

Drowsiness

See BILIOUSNESS.

Dysentery (Bloody stools)

Inflammation of the mucous membrane of the large bowel or colon. Passages of stool are small, difficult, and frequent, with much crampy pain. Stools consist mainly of mucus tinged with blood. The abdomen is hard, but tender along the colon. The skin is hot, the thirst is excessive, the appetite poor. Vomiting and fever are often present. Rest in bed and the application of heat to the abdomen are advisable. A warm flannel bandage should be worn around the abdomen at all times. Only warm drinks should be given. The diet should be light and nonirritating. Foods that are slimy when cooked, such as barley, rice, sago, and other starchy mixtures, are beneficial. Fruit and raw foods should be avoided.

Remedies: Use No. 39 in conjunction with No. 35.

Assisting the Treatment: To be used in conjunction with the foregoing: In dyspepsia, use No. 93. Where a general tonic might be of benefit, No. 11 should be taken.

Dyspepsia
See STOMACH DISORDERS.

Earache
Shooting, gnawing pains in the ear are generally caused by colds in the head, nose, or throat; they are also often due to neuralgia, rheumatism, influenza, or inflammation in the ear itself. In the latter instance there may also be a discharge from the ear. High blood pressure may also cause ear troubles. (See BLOOD PRESSURE, HIGH.)

Applications to the ear of hot compresses made from an infusion of chamomile flowers or hops will be found very beneficial and at the same time will help to relieve the pain. To act as a local antiseptic, No. 40 should be used.

Remedy: Use No. 40, as noted above.

Assisting the Treatment: To be used in conjunction with No. 40: In case of cold or influenza, use No. 20. In case of neuralgia, use No. 72. In case of rheumatism, use Nos. 83 and 84. In case of nervousness, use No. 66 or 67 or 68.

Ear Noises
See BLOOD PRESSURE, HIGH; EARACHE; NERVOUSNESS; "Symptoms," p. 25.

Ear Wax
See EARACHE. Use No. 40.

Eczema (Salt rheum or tetter)
Eczema is a collective name for a variety of skin eruptions and appears in different forms. Often at first only but an annoying itching is noticed, but soon the skin becomes reddened and more or less inflamed. Dry or wet blotches appear, often of a scaly or crusty

nature, sometimes in the form of small blisters or pimples containing a watery secretion or pus. The cause of these eruptions can generally be traced to poor circulation of the blood, constipation, dyspepsia, sluggishness of the liver or kidneys, nervous debility, or other forms of constitutional derangements, which gradually result in an accumulation of impurities in the blood. It is therefore self-evident that all efforts to correct the trouble must be directed toward removing the underlying cause. A preparation acting as a depurative, or blood purifier, should be used in all cases. External remedies should be used to relieve the itching and to induce healing. Water should be kept away from eczema as much as possible.

Remedies: Internally, use either No. 54 or 55, in all cases. For dry eczema, use externally No. 41.

Assisting the Treatment: To be used in conjunction with the above: In stomach disorders, use No. 90 or 91. In nervous debility, use No. 92 or 93.

Edema
See DROPSY.

Enema (Internal bath; colon flush)
For the internal bath, or enema, chemicals or other irritating matter should not be used to remove hardened, encrusted, or decayed matter from the colon. Substances used should by all means be mild, yet possess properties that act as a cleansing agent upon the lining of the bowels without being irritating. Herbs, properly used and selected, should not have an irritating effect; rather than weaken the delicate tissues, herbs should help give them tone and cleanse them without doing any harm.

Remedy: No. 42 is a well-tried and effective remedy.

Epilepsy
In this disease, the nerve-quieting effect of certain herbs has often given relief. Intestinal worms sometimes bring on such attacks; it is therefore advisable to watch the stools in such cases. The diet should be light, and the food should be chewed slowly and well. Overloading

the stomach and fast eating usually bring on indigestion, which will aggravate this condition. In fact, indigestion is often responsible for this trouble.

[There are many other causes for convulsive disorders, and medical attention should be sought to rule out serious conditions.]

Remedy: Use No. 43.

Assisting the Treatment: To be used in conjunction with No. 43: In worms, use No. 102. In indigestion, use No. 92 or 93. In nervousness, use No. 68.

Eyes, Inflamed, Weak, and Tired

This condition is generally due to colds, strain, overwork, the presence of foreign matter, or deranged conditions of the system. The cause, of course, must first be removed.

Remedy: No. 44 will be found effective and reliable, and can be used with perfect safety in all such cases of eye trouble.

Assisting the Treatment: To be used in conjunction with No. 44: If the system is run-down, use No. 11. In nervousness, use No. 66 or 68.

Face Ache

See NEURALGIA.

Fainting Spells

Remedy: Smelling Salts, No. 70.

Falling Out of Hair

See DANDRUFF.

Feet, Sweating, Burning, Sore

Excessive sweating of the feet is an abnormal condition and should be reduced to a more normal degree, without, however, suppressing it entirely. Sweating is nature's way to rid the system of acids and other impurities, the retention of which might lead to more serious troubles in some other part of the body.

Remedies: Use No. 45 as a dusting powder, and No. 46 as a wash.

Assisting the Treatment: To be used in conjunction with the above: If the bowels are not properly regulated, use No. 54 or 55.

Felon
See WHITLOW OF THE FINGER.

Female Disorders
See MENSTRUATION.

Fever
See COLD OR ACUTE CATARRH OF THE HEAD.

Fever Blisters
Remedy: Healing Balsam, No. 89.

Flatulence
See STOMACH DISORDERS.

Flushes Toward the Head
See MENOPAUSE; DYSPEPSIA.

Frequent Urination
See BLADDER, INFLAMMATION OF; also DIABETES.

Frostbite
See CHILBLAINS.

Fullness in the Head
See BLOOD PRESSURE, HIGH.

Fullness in the Stomach
See STOMACH DISORDERS.

Gallbladder, Inflammation of
This trouble may originate with exposure to cold or wet, with continuous excesses in eating and drinking, or with infection of the

gallbladder and its duct by germs. A catarrhal inflammation of the mucosa and swelling gradually set in, and the duct leading from the gallbladder becomes partially or entirely obstructed by catarrhal slime, congealed bile, or gallstones. The bile, being thus retained, is forced back into the liver, and from there enters the blood, coloring the blood and the skin more or less yellow, and is finally expelled through the urine. Such urine is of a dark amber or reddish color, heavy, and loaded with urates and bile matter.

The pain caused by this condition is especially noticed on the right side, below the lowest rib, often extending backward toward the shoulder blade, or across the stomach, often creating the impression that the trouble is in the stomach. This impression is often correct, as the stomach may also be affected by the catarrhal inflammation.

The bowels as a rule are constipated, and the stool at times whitish-gray or clay-colored. The skin is yellow and dry and often itchy. The tongue is coated, the appetite poor, and nausea and vomiting of a yellowish-green slime may occur. The stomach is generally very much upset. In fact, the inflammation in the gallbladder and its ducts may originate with a catarrhal condition in the stomach.

Treatment: The diet should be light and should be mainly composed of plainly cooked vegetables, ripe fruits, and salads with a simple dressing of olive oil with a dash of lemon juice. Starches should be eaten in moderation. This also applies to meats, which should be lean, and preferably the so-called "white meats," such as chicken and fish. Meats should be either boiled or broiled, never fried. Sweets, greasy foods, and fats, including butter, should be avoided. Rest and sunshine are beneficial. In order to improve the function of the affected organs, proper regulation of stomach, liver, and bowels must be accomplished.

Remedies: Use Nos. 47 and 48.

Assisting the Treatment: To be used in conjunction with the above: In stomach disorders, use No. 90 or 92 or 93.

Gallstones
See GALLBLADDER, INFLAMMATION OF.

Gas in the Stomach
See STOMACH DISORDERS; BILIOUSNESS.

Gastritis
See STOMACH DISORDERS.

Glands, Swollen
See TONSILLITIS.

Gout
Defective elimination and sluggishness of the whole system, due to lack of exercise, high living, and errors in diet, are all contributing factors in this rheumatic condition, which arises from excess uric acid in the body fluids.

To overcome this condition, it is necessary to improve the activity of the vital organs and cause better elimination of waste products from the system. The diet should consist mostly of vegetable matter. Meats, starches, and sweets should be used only moderately. Alcoholic drinks should be avoided. Perspiration is beneficial and should be encouraged from time to time, by using No. 21 or 22, and by taking an occasional steam bath. Cold compresses, especially if made with an herb vinegar (see No. 52) and applied to the affected part, will tend to relieve the pain and fever.

Remedy: Use No. 51.

Assisting the Treatment: To be used in conjunction with the above: In stomach disorders, use No. 90 or 92. To improve the blood, use No. 54 or 55.

Granulated Eyelids
See EYES.

Gravel in the Urine
See STONES OR GRAVEL IN KIDNEYS OR BLADDER.

Grippe
See COLD OR ACUTE CATARRH IN THE HEAD.

Gums, Sore, Bleeding, or Spongy

This trouble may accompany a disordered stomach or constipation. The underlying cause should, therefore, be corrected first. The mouth should be thoroughly rinsed three to four times a day with a decoction made from No. 98. Teeth should be brushed and cleaned with dental floss regularly to remove bacteria-promoting food residue from around the teeth.

[Prolonged and intractable cases of bleeding gums should receive medical attention, since this may be a symptom of a more serious underlying condition.]

Assisting the Treatment: To be used in conjunction with No. 98: In stomach disorders, use No. 90 or 92. In constipation, use No. 26 or 27. For impure blood, use No. 54 or 55.

Hair, Falling Out of

See DANDRUFF.

Hardening of the Arteries

See BLOOD PRESSURE, HIGH.

Hardness of Hearing

See COLD OR ACUTE CATARRH IN THE HEAD; EARACHE; NASAL CATARRH.

Hay Fever (Summer catarrh)

This seasonal allergic inflammation of the nasal and bronchial mucous membrane should be treated the same as chronic nasal catarrh.

Remedy: Use No. 64.

Assisting the Treatment: To be used in conjunction with No. 64: In nervous irritability, use No. 68. In run-down condition, use No. 11. If constipated, use No. 26 or 27.

Headache

This is not a disease in itself, but the result of an underlying disturbance in some part of the body. Keeping this in mind, it is obvious that headaches cannot be cured by simply suppressing the symptom—pain—and allowing the underlying cause to keep existing. That is precisely what happens when strong chemicals are taken to relieve a headache. Headaches are often caused by disorders of the stomach, biliousness, constipation, menstrual irregularities, overwork, deficiency of the blood, high blood pressure, eyestrain, and disturbances of the lungs and heart, as well as by infections or structural abnormalities (masses, blood clots, etc.) affecting the head and brain proper.

There are natural remedies in this book for various disturbances that may be responsible for a headache. Make use of them. Get at the root of the trouble by removing the cause. Do not be satisfied with temporary relief. Headache remedies will give only temporary relief, and will in the long run harm the system.

Remedies: In stomach disorders, use No. 90 or 91. In constipation, use No. 26 or 27. In menstrual irregularities, use No. 60 or 61 or 62. In nasal catarrh, use Nos. 20 and 64. In high blood pressure, use No. 9 or 10. In nervousness, use No. 92 or 93. In biliousness, use No. 6 or 25.

Healing Balsam

See No. 89.

Hearing, Hardness of

See COLD OR ACUTE CATARRH IN THE HEAD; EARACHE; NASAL CATARRH.

Heartburn

See STOMACH DISORDERS.

Hemorrhoids (Piles)

Hemorrhoids are enlargements of the veins in the rectum. They owe their existence to a stagnation of the blood in the abdominal venous system and to pressure from straining to pass hard and dry stools. The veins become gradually distended, and piles are the result. They are filled with blood and at times are very painful and itchy (itching hemorrhoids). Pressure or friction may cause them to burst and bleed (bleeding hemorrhoids). When they protrude, they are called "external hemorrhoids."

Pressure in the rectum is often responsible for all these troubles, and in order to correct them, the bowels must be kept well regulated. It is advisable, however, not to use strong medicines, as their irritating action will cause the hemorrhoids to become more inflamed, sore, and painful.

Remedies: Use No. 76 to keep the bowels regulated. No. 77 should be used as a rectal wash, and No. 78, which is a healing suppository, should be inserted in the rectum every night before retiring, and allowed to stay there overnight.

Assisting the Treatment: Hot sitz baths, if piles are not bleeding, or if the patient is not very strong. (See SITZ BATHS, HOT.) Cold sitz baths, when an inflamed condition prevails and the patient is strong. (See SITZ BATHS, COLD.)

High Blood Pressure
See BLOOD PRESSURE, HIGH.

Hives (Nettle rash)
This allergic rash may be due to insect bites, specific substances, or foods to which the individual is sensitive, such as unripe fruits, fat pork, crabmeat, fish, oysters, pickles, etc.

Whitish or reddish elevated spots (wheals) appear on the skin, accompanied by a tingling, itching sensation. Headache or slight fever may be present.

Treatment: In order to remove the irritating food or poisonous matter that is responsible for the condition, the bowels should be kept open and the blood cleaned by using No. 54 or 55. The diet should be light and non-irritating. The foods responsible for the trouble should be eliminated from one's diet. Hot baths, with the water softened by adding a handful of borax, and washing or sponging with extract of witch hazel or alcohol are very beneficial.

Assisting the Treatment: In stomach disorders, use No. 90 or 91, in conjunction with the above.

Hoarseness (Loss of voice)

This disturbance may be due to a weakness and swelling of the vocal cords from overstraining or from cold and coughs, or to an infection of the larynx. Chronic hoarseness should be investigated medically, since it may be a symptom of a serious underlying condition.

Remedy: Use No. 53.

Assisting the Treatment: In colds, use Nos. 20 and 98 in conjunction with No. 53. In bronchitis, use No. 14 or 15.

Impotence

See SEXUAL WEAKNESS.

Impure Blood

Poor action of liver and bowels, a faulty digestion, or disturbances in the lymphatic glands are generally responsible for the accumulation of impurities in the blood. Eruptions of the skin in the form of abscesses, pimples (acne), boils, blackheads, and a sallow complexion are the result.

Remedies: Use No. 54 or 55.

Assisting the Treatment: To be used in conjunction with the above: If stomach does not function properly, use No. 90. In nervous disorders, use No. 92.

Indigestion

See STOMACH DISORDERS.

Inflammation of the Bladder

See BLADDER, INFLAMMATION OR CATARRH OF OF.

Inflammation of the Bowels

See DIARRHEA.

Inflammation of the Gallbladder

See GALLBLADDER, INFLAMMATION OF.

Inflammation of the Kidneys
See KIDNEYS, INFLAMMATION OF.

Inflammation of the Stomach
See STOMACH DISORDERS.

Inflammation of the Throat
See TONSILLITIS.

Influenza
See COLD OR ACUTE CATARRH IN THE HEAD.

Insomnia
See SLEEPLESSNESS; NERVOUSNESS.

Internal Bath
See ENEMA.

Irregular Menses
See MENSTRUATION, IRREGULAR, SCANTY, OR SUPPRESSED.

Itching of the Skin
See ECZEMA; LICE; SCABIES; BILIOUSNESS; HIVES; DIABETES; MEASLES; also "Symptoms," p. 24.

Jaundice
See BILIOUSNESS; GALLBLADDER, INFLAMMATION OF.

Kidneys, Inflammation of (Nephritis)
This trouble generally begins with a chilly sensation followed by fever, headache, and pain in the small of the back. The skin is pale and dry, and heart action slow and forcible. The urine is scanty, deep amber colored, strong in odor, leaving a heavy sediment upon standing. It is sometimes mixed with blood. Albumin is generally found in the urine. Swelling of the face, eyelids, ankles, and other parts of

the body may appear later if the trouble is neglected. The disease may become chronic and more dangerous.

The diet should consist mostly of vegetable matter, with meats, eggs, starches, and sweets used very sparingly.

Remedy: Use No. 57.

Assisting the Treatment: To be used in conjunction with the above: If liver is sluggish, use No. 6. If constipated, use No. 26 or 27 instead of No. 6.

Kidneys, Stones or Gravel In
See STONES OR GRAVEL IN KIDNEYS OR BLADDER.

Lameness
See RHEUMATISM.

Leukorrhea
A catarrhal inflammation of the mucous membrane lining of the vagina, cervix, or uterus, with a discharge of a whitish or yellowish fluid. Some mucus discharge is normal at times in all women, but prolonged or excessive discharge of an irritating character may be a sign of infection. Strong, irritating medicines should be avoided as they act as irritants and tend to destroy the delicate tissues. Warm sitz baths are very beneficial.

Remedy: Use No. 58.

Assisting the Treatment: To be used in conjunction with the above: If due to general weakness, use No. 11. If due to impure blood, use No. 54 or 55. If constipated, use No. 26 or 27.

Liniment
See No. 84.

Liver, Congestion of
See BILIOUSNESS; CONSTIPATION.

Liver, Torpid and Sluggish
See BILIOUSNESS; CONSTIPATION.

Loss of Voice
See HOARSENESS.

Lumbago
See RHEUMATISM.

Measles
Generally begins with a light cold, mild cough, and slight fever. The tongue is coated and the throat and nasal passages show catarrhal inflammation. After the fourth day, numerous irregular, elevated, dark red spots appear on the face, gradually extending to the neck and down the trunk to the lower extremities, attended by an itching or burning sensation. This condition exists from three to five days, then the eruptions begin to fade and peel off in bran-like scales.

Although this disease is usually comparatively harmless, it may cause serious complications if neglected, and therefore should always receive proper attention. By all means, the patient should be kept in bed, and on a light diet.

Remedy: Use No. 59.

Assisting the Treatment: To be used in conjunction with the above: If constipated, use No. 28. If pores are not open, use No. 22. To relieve itching, apply Healing Balsam No. 89.

Menopause (Change of life)
Great help in the disturbances that occur during this critical period of life in women is obtained from herb combination No. 18. It tends to relieve the symptoms accompanying menopause, including hot flushes, dizziness, headache, pain in the pelvis and back, and general weakness.

Remedy: No. 18.

Assisting the Treatment: To be used in conjunction with No. 18: If nervous, use No. 66 or 67 or 68. If constipated and bilious, use No. 6 or 26 or 27. In stomach disorders, use No. 90 or 91 or 92 or 93. In general weakness, use No. 11.

Menstruation, Irregular, Scanty, or Suppressed

This condition is generally brought on by exposure to cold or wet, poor conditions of the blood, nervousness, or violent emotions. It is essential that the underlying cause be removed and the general tone of the system increased.

Remedy: Use No. 60.

Assisting the Treatment: To be used in conjunction with the above: If due to nervous disturbances, use No. 68. If blood is impoverished, use No. 11. If a blood purifier is needed, use No. 54 or 55.

Menstruation, Painful and Spasmodic

This may be due to inflammation or obstructions, or other problems in the uterus. Pain can be aggravated by emotional and psychic factors.

Remedy: Use No. 61.

Menstruation, Profuse

Excessive menstrual flow is generally preceded by pain and weakness in the low midback. Some women are predisposed to uterine hemorrhages due to a flabby or relaxed texture of the uterus. Other contributing factors include overexercise, heavy lifting, injuries, or mental excitement. If it persists too long, it may cause general weakness, a sallow, unhealthy complexion, headaches, and nervous debility. In persistent profuse menstruation, the cause should be identified through medical investigation and corrected.

Remedy: Use No. 62.

Assisting the Treatment: To be used in conjunction with the above: If constipated, use No. 26 or 27. In nervous weakness, use No. 68.

Moths

No. 63 will keep them out of closets and dressers.

Muscular Rheumatism

See RHEUMATISM.

Nail Biting
See BITING THE FINGERNAILS.

Nasal Catarrh (Catarrh in the head)
Repeated attacks of acute catarrh, or nasal mucous membrane inflammation (see COLD), may gradually result in a chronic form of the disease, commonly known as catarrh in the head, or simply catarrh. A continuous discharge of mucus takes place and the air passages are more or less obstructed all the time.

Remedies: Use No. 64 or 65.

Assisting the Treatment: To be taken in conjunction with the above: If constipated, or if a blood purifier is needed, use No. 54 or 55.

Nausea
See STOMACH DISORDERS.

Neck, Stiff
See RHEUMATISM; also No. 84.

Nephritis
See KIDNEYS, INFLAMMATION OF.

Nerve Pain
See NEURALGIA; NEURITIS; SCIATICA.

Nervous Dyspepsia
See STOMACH DISORDERS.

Nervous Exhaustion
See NERVOUSNESS.

Nervous Headache
See STOMACH DISORDERS; DYSPEPSIA.

Nervous Indigestion

See STOMACH DISORDERS; DYSPEPSIA.

Nervous Weakness

See NERVOUSNESS.

Nervousness

A condition of exhaustion due to overtaxing the powers of body and mind. Overwork, worry, excitement, loss of sleep, excesses in eating and drinking, undue strain on the vital forces and nerve centers are generally responsible for the irritability and weakness of the nervous system.

In order to improve this condition, it is self-evident that the underlying cause must be removed and the building up of the nervous system's forces instituted, by avoiding excesses of any kind. Rest, fresh air, sunshine, pleasant thoughts and surroundings, wholesome simple foods are not only beneficial but essential. Coffee and tea should be avoided, as they irritate the nervous system. They are often responsible for restlessness and sleeplessness at night and irritability in the daytime.

The following herbal recipes will be found very beneficial.

Remedies: Use No. 66 or 67 or 68 or 69 or 70 or 71.

Assisting the Treatment: In nervous dyspepsia, use No. 92 or 93. In nervous headache, use No. 6. As a general tonic, use No. 11. As a substitute for coffee or tea, use No. 71, or maté leaves.

Nettle Rash

See HIVES.

Neuralgia

A nervous disorder characterized by a darting, boring, or stabbing pain extending along the course of a nerve or its branches. The pain is more generally confined to the head (face ache), but may also affect other parts of the body. (See SCIATICA and NEURITIS.) Exposure to cold and draft, derangement of the digestive organs or the blood, nerve pressure, and decayed teeth are among the factors responsible for the trouble.

Since many cases of neuralgia are accompanied by incomplete elimination of waste products from the system and the resulting impoverishment of the blood, special attention should be paid to the proper functions of stomach, liver, and bowels.

Remedy: Use externally No. 72.

Assisting the Treatment: In stomach disorders, use No. 90 or 92 or 93. In constipation or impure blood, use No. 54 or 55. In nervous disturbances, use No. 66 or 68.

Neuritis

A painful inflammation of one or several nerves, brought on by exposure to cold or wet, nerve pressure, injuries, stretching of nerves, and the accumulation of morbid matter in the system. It is also often observed, as an after-effect, in rheumatism, gout, syphilis, and diabetes. The underlying cause must be treated in order to obtain results in this disease.

Remedy: Use No. 73.

Assisting the Treatment: In rheumatism, use No. 84. In constipation or impure blood, use No. 54 or 55. In biliousness, use No. 6 instead of No. 54 or 55.

Night Sweats

The abnormal secretion of the sweat glands in certain diseases can only be explained as the self-aid of nature to eliminate morbid matter from the system. Accordingly, night sweats should not be suppressed entirely. However, if continuous sweating should have a weakening effect on the system, No. 74 may be used without any harmful effect.

Remedy: Use No. 74.

Assisting the Treatment: In case of bodily weakness, use No. 11. In case of nervous weakness, use No. 68.

Nipples, Sore

Remedy: HEALING BALSAM, No. 89.

Numbness
See COLD FEET AND HANDS.

Obesity
Lack of exercise and overeating of fat-producing foods (starches, sugars, fats) are generally responsible for this trouble. It is therefore advisable to live more on a vegetable diet and to eat plenty of ripe fruits. Moderate daily exercise should be engaged in, and a hot sweat bath or, still better, a steam bath, may be taken once or twice a week. The frequency of these baths should be regulated in accordance with one's constitution. Proper elimination through the bowels should be maintained. Dulse or kelp, taken in small quantities daily, will supply the element iodine in a natural form, which acts as a normalizer.

You will find the following recipe well balanced as to its eliminative and normalizing properties, and it is therefore an excellent aid in the treatment of obesity.

Remedy: Use No. 75.

Offensive Breath
See STOMACH DISORDERS. Where the condition is due to neglect of oral hygiene, use No. 98 as a prophylactic.

Offensive Sweating
See BODY ODOR.

Pain in the Abdomen
See "Symptoms," p. 23.

Pain in the Back
See "Symptoms," p. 22.

Pain in the Bladder
See "Symptoms," p. 23.

Pain in the Chest
See "Symptoms," p. 22.

Pain in the Head
See "Symptoms," p. 21.

Pain in the Neck
See NEURITIS; NEURALGIA; NERVOUSNESS.

Pain in the Pelvis
See "Symptoms," p. 22.

Pain in the Rectum
See "Symptoms," p. 23.

Pain in the Stomach
See "Symptoms," p. 22.

Pain in the Throat
See "Symptoms," p. 23.

Painful Menstruation
See MENSTRUATION, PAINFUL.

Painful Urination
See BLADDER, INFLAMMATION OF.

Perspiration, Offensive
See BODY ODOR.

Piles
See HEMORRHOIDS.

Pimples
See IMPURE BLOOD.

Pimples, Inflamed
See BOILS AND INFLAMED PIMPLES.

Pinworms

See WORMS.

Pleurisy

An inflammation of the membrane covering the lungs and lining of the internal surface of the chest. It begins generally with shivering and chills, or slight fever, followed by a sharp and cutting pain in the chest, especially when taking a deep breath. Unforeseen motion, coughing, and sneezing bring on and increase the pain and make breathing more difficult. This condition may lead to serious consequences if neglected. The patient should be placed in bed, in a well-ventilated, warm room. The diet should be light. The bowels should be well regulated. Application of hot compresses or poultices is beneficial. Perspiration should be induced. Care should be taken that the night clothes are dry and the patient kept warm.

Remedy: Use No. 79.

Assisting the Treatment: Application of hot towels or poultice, No. 82, to the chest, or rubbing in of liniment, No. 84. The chest should be thoroughly dried before applying the liniment.

To induce perspiration, use No. 21 or 22. If constipated, use No. 26 or 27. In bronchitis, use No. 14 or 15.

Podagra

See GOUT.

Poison Oak and Poison Ivy

Inflammation of the skin due to the poisonous effect of the poison oak or poison ivy plant. Swelling, burning, and itching of the affected parts and sometimes the appearance of innumerable small blisters characterize the infection.

Some people are more susceptible to this poisoning than others, possibly due to their comparative lack of resistance; because of the sluggish condition of their systems, they are not able to counteract and eliminate the poisonous substances they come in contact with.

The treatment should be both external and internal. The internal remedies should be such as to promote a better function of the stomach, liver, and bowels. The external application should be of a soothing nature.

Remedy: Use No. 80.

Assisting the Treatment: If constipated, or if blood is out of order, use No. 54 or 55. If stomach is out of order, use No. 90 or 92.

Profuse Menstruation
See MENSTRUATION, PROFUSE.

Quinsy
See TONSILLITIS.

Rash
See ECZEMA; HIVES.

Rheumatism
Incomplete elimination of waste products created by decomposed food and poisonous matter, decayed teeth or tonsils, exposure to cold or dampness, and hereditary predisposition are among the conditions responsible for rheumatic disorders.

The disease manifests itself in many ways; the underlying cause, however, seems to be the same, namely the accumulation of excessive amounts of decomposition products, especially in the form of uric acid in the blood. This substance, when not eliminated, is carried by the blood through the entire system and deposited in the tissues of the organs, where the circulation is the poorest, causing inflammation and pain or forming deposits. The particular form of rheumatism is named for the part affected. Thus, if the inner linings of the arteries, veins, or joints are affected, it is called "articular rheumatism" or arteritis; if the muscles are affected, muscular rheumatism; if the nerves are affected, it is named sciatica, neuritis, or neuralgia; if the lumbar region is affected, it is called lumbago. If the small joints of the hands and feet are affected, it is termed gout.

Treatment should include a thorough cleaning of the whole system and the promotion of better elimination of waste matter. Sciatica, neuralgia, and neuritis are rheumatic conditions affecting certain nerves. These are not considered here, but under their respective headings.

A light and, if possible, purely vegetable diet should be resorted to for some time. If there is no desire for food, a fast of two to three days is advisable, during which time plain water with the possible addition of fruit juices should be used freely.

Remedies: To aid the processes of elimination, it is advisable to use daily No. 83. To aid the circulation in the parts affected, use liniment No. 84 before retiring. To further aid the elimination processes through the pores of the skin (sweating), use No. 21 or 22 once or twice a week, depending upon one's constitution.

Assisting the Treatment: If tonsils are affected, gargle several times a day with No. 98. If the stomach is out of order, use No. 90 or 92. In lumbago, hot sitz baths should be taken before retiring. (see SITZ BATHS, HOT).

Ringing in the Ears

See EARACHE; BLOOD PRESSURE, HIGH; "Symptoms," p. 25.

Running of the Ear

See EARACHE.

Salt Rheum

See ECZEMA.

Scabies (Itch)

A contagious disease due to the invasion of the skin by microscopically small animal parasites. The rash caused by the insects consists of small blisters filled with a watery liquid; the itching is intense and more noticeable at night. Scratching increases the soreness and itching.

Remedy: Use No. 56.

Scalds

See SKIN, ROUGH CHAPPED OR CRACKED; WOUNDS.

Scalp Disease

See ECZEMA; DANDRUFF.

Sciatica

A rheumatic condition affecting the sciatic nerve, which extends along the back part of the thigh, down to the calf of the leg, and to the sole of the foot. Sciatica is characterized by a gnawing, sometimes very severe pain, following the course of the nerve or its branches, but may also affect only a part of it. This trouble is closely related to neuritis; in fact, it is generally the result of it. Sciatica may therefore be treated like neuritis. (See NEURITIS.)

Sexual Weakness (Impotence)

In this trouble, it is absolutely necessary to build up the general health and invigorate the nervous system, which supplies strength and vitality to the weakened organs. Excesses that led to the trouble must be avoided. The diet should be composed of wholesome, plain, non-irritating food, and a quiet, restful life is necessary to allow the system to recuperate and revitalize itself.

Hot and cold compresses applied alternately over the lumbar region before retiring are very beneficial, as they tend to stimulate the nerves of the second and third lumbar vertebrae, which control the weakened organs.

Some herbs have a tonic action upon the glands; if used for a while, in conjunction with the proper rest of body and mind, they should give good results. In No. 86, the most effective herbs have been combined in the right proportions. These herbs are extensively used, with apparent success, in the countries of their origin.

Remedy: Use No. 86.

Assisting the Treatment: To be used in conjunction with the above: In bodily weakness, use No. 11. In nervous exhaustion, use No. 68. Cold sitz baths should be taken several times a week, always before retiring (see SITZ BATHS, COLD).

Shingles

A skin eruption generally spreading across the breast or waist, like a belt, on one side of the body, following the course of a nerve. The skin is reddened, and along the affected nerve a vesicular rash appears that, if properly treated, dries into a yellowish-brown crust upon the skin after a week or two and then drops off.

Chills, fever, and pain along the affected nerves generally precede the foregoing symptoms. It is essential to keep the stomach, liver, and bowels well regulated. The inflammation and pain may be relieved by the use of a dusting powder (see No. 87), which will tend to hasten the healing process and assist in drying up the crusts.

Remedies: Use No. 87 as a dusting powder. No. 88 should be used as a compress. No. 89 should be used as an ointment when necessary.

Assisting the Treatment: In stomach disorders, use No. 92 or 93. In constipation, use No. 26 or 27. In case of sluggish liver, use No. 6.

Shortness of Breath
See "Symptoms," p. 25.

Sick Headache
See BILIOUSNESS.

Sinking Spells
See FAINTING SPELLS; NERVOUSNESS.

Sitz Bath, Hot
Where a regular sitz bathtub is not available, an ordinary old-fashioned galvanized washtub will do. Fill the tub one-third full with warm water and let the patient sit in it, submerging only the lower portion of the body, leaving the feet and upper part of the body out of the water. Add warmer water from time to time, gradually making it as hot as can be comfortably tolerated. A blanket may be used to cover the upper part of the body, and the bath may be extended to fifteen or twenty minutes. This bath is especially indicated in suppressed and painful urination and suppressed and painful menstruation, gravel in the bladder, rheumatism, lumbago, and other inflammatory affections. The addition of certain herbs, such as watermint,

chamomile, oat straw, pine needles, etc., makes this bath still more effective.

Sitz Bath, Cold
The cold sitz bath is taken in the same way as the hot sitz bath, with the exception that cold water is used and it should only last from 1 to 3 minutes. The bath is used for its tonic effect in cases of relaxed tissues of the pelvis; in abdominal, sexual, and intestinal complaints, in hemorrhoids, and in constipation.

Skin Eruptions
See ECZEMA; SKIN, ROUGH, CHAPPED, OR CRACKED.

Skin, Rough, Chapped, or Cracked
Remedy: No. 89.

Sleeplessness
Remedy: No. 85. See also NERVOUSNESS.

Sores, Open
See WOUNDS.
Remedies: See No. 89 or 13 or 103.

Sores, Ulcerated or Discharging
See BOILS AND INFLAMED PIMPLES.

Sore Throat
See TONSILLITIS.

Sour Stomach
See STOMACH DISORDERS.

Sprains
Remedy: No. 84.

Stiffness in Neck, Limbs, and Muscles
See RHEUMATISM.

Stomach Disorders

Several different diseases fall under this heading, but the direct cause of almost all of them is the same: Fast eating, not chewing the food properly, overloading, and not eating the right kind of food are generally responsible for the troubles. The bad habits must be abandoned in order to effect a cure, as there is no medicine that can chew the food properly, or stop anybody from overeating, or prevent one from eating things that are hard to digest.

Food that is not properly masticated is retained longer in the stomach than it should be. As a result, it turns sour and ferments, and creates an excessive amount of acid and gas. This in turn causes a great deal of irritation and inflammation of the mucous lining of the whole digestive tract. A catarrhal condition gradually sets in; the lining becomes coated with a thick, slimy mucus that interferes with the assimilation of the food. Decomposition and decay are the result, and poisonous matter therefrom is absorbed, which leads to severe disturbances of the stomach and bowels and gradually of the whole system. The result of this is far-reaching, as it finally leads to many other diseases to which the human race is heir. It is therefore only too true that "most people dig their own graves with their teeth."

Let us therefore repeat what we might call the Golden Rule of Health: Eat slowly, chew your food well, and DON'T OVERLOAD. Eat only plain food, plenty of fresh vegetables, salads, and ripe fruits. The richer foods, such as meats, eggs, starches, sweets, etc., should be taken more moderately and only in proportion to one's degree of daily physical exertion. In that way the food can be balanced properly and the digestion can go on more completely. Failure to live up to these simple, natural rules will gradually lead to the operating table, but the operation will not remove the underlying cause, and consequently will not bring the desired relief.

Catarrh of the Stomach (Gastritis; chronic dyspepsia)

An inflamed condition of the mucous lining of the stomach generally brought on by continuous abuse of food and drink. Incomplete mastication, overloading the stomach with food or drink that is too hot or too cold, food that is too fat or hard to digest, the excessive use of liquor, coffee, tea, and tobacco are mostly responsible for the trouble. Gastritis first starts in an acute attack, but gradually becomes chronic if neglected, and the attacks become more frequent and consequently harder to cure.

Shortly after eating, but sometimes an hour or two afterward, a feeling of fullness and heaviness is noticed in the region of the stomach, with nausea, belching, and eructations of sour, often fermented food. The appetite is diminished, and there is an aversion generally to those things that may be responsible for the attack, while at the same time there may be a strong desire for spicy, sour, or salty foods.

In adults, constipation generally prevails, while children suffer more often from diarrhea. The tongue is usually coated, and heartburn, dizziness, and palpitations of the heart may be present. The region of the stomach is tender and sensitive to pressure. If there is an inclination to vomiting, it should be induced by filling the stomach with warm water and tickling the palate with the finger until the desired effect is accomplished. For a day or two, the diet should consist of soups, especially those that cook slimy, like barley, rice, sago, or farina, with stale bread or zwieback. Gradually more nourishing but light food may be added.

If no desire for food exists, a fast of a day or two is advisable, but drinking of fresh, clean water in small quantities should always be allowed. In case of cramps and pain in the stomach, apply hot steam compresses to that region; in case of heat and fever, cold, wet compresses should be used instead.

Remedies: Use No. 90 or 91.

Assisting the Treatment: If constipated, use No. 26 or 27; but if liver is sluggish, use No. 6 instead. In anemia, use No. 11.

Dyspepsia (Heartburn; indigestion; nervous dyspepsia)

There is a great similarity in the symptoms of nervous dyspepsia and those of chronic catarrh of the stomach, yet there is a decided difference between the causes of the two ailments.

In chronic catarrh of the stomach, there is an inflamed condition of the membrane of the stomach, which causes anatomical changes in the lining of the stomach; nervous dyspepsia is due almost entirely to disturbances in the nervous system that controls the stomach, with no such changes of the mucous lining taking place.

The stomach has a network of nerves, which is controlled by nerve centers of the brain. This nerve system in the stomach is very sensitive and can react to the slightest provocation. If abused, it causes digestive disturbances that retard and disarrange the functions of the entire digestive tract. It may even produce pain in the stomach. This condition is very often brought about through overwork, worry, mental excitement, grief, fear, despondency, overeating, lack of exercise, and among other things, too rich or too unbalanced a diet.

There is often a sense of fullness, although the stomach may be empty. Gas pressure, heartburn, nausea, rumbling in the stomach due to flatulence, spitting up of partly digested food or sour liquid, and pain or soreness at the pit of the stomach during digestion may also be present. Belching sometimes affords temporary relief, as may eating, but the basic condition is not improved by taking in more food, since it only tends to form more gas. Palpitations of the heart, headache, dizziness, and flushes toward the head are often experienced. The bowels are generally constipated, the tongue soft and flabby, and the urine scanty. Restlessness and even sleeplessness at night may also occur. For days a normal condition may exist, but all of a sudden a feeling of despondency may appear and even the lightest kind of food may cause distress.

A prescribed diet will often result in failure, as each individual must study his or her own diet. We are not all alike and what is good food for one may not agree with another. Food that seemingly does not distress at one meal may do so at the next. It is, however, advisable to select easily digestible foods, such as softboiled or raw eggs, underdone meats, green vegetables, broth thickened with barley, oatmeal, sago, rice, or farina, and other such foods the patient knows agree with him or her. Instead of coffee or tea, herb tea No. 71, or peppermint or linden flower tea should be used, as they aid the digestion and do not irritate the nerves that control the stomach as coffee and ordinary tea do.

Remedies: Use No. 92 or 93.

Assisting the Treatment: If constipated, use No. 26 or 27; but if bilious, then use No. 6 instead. In nervous weakness, use No. 68.

Ulcer of the Stomach and Duodenum

When, through continuous attacks of indigestion, the mucous lining of the stomach becomes weakened and the blood supply diminished, the mucous membrane, not being sufficiently nourished, loses its resistance and becomes open to attack by the acid juices of the stomach; then ulcers may form. Excessive amounts of acid formed by a faulty digestion gradually lead to the destruction of the lining and the development of ulcers. When a blood vessel becomes destroyed by an ulcer, bleeding, or hemorrhage, takes place. The blood, if vomited, is of a bright red color, but if passed through the bowels, it generally appears in the stools as a dark, tarry substance. (In case of cancer of the stomach, the vomit often has the appearance of coffee grounds.)

Food vomited up is undigested, very sour and slimy. Spasmodic, gnawing pains are felt from time to time in the pit of the stomach and, not infrequently, the pain is felt in the back, between the shoulder blades. The pain is generally relieved by eating. The stomach is quite sensitive to pressure, and easily irritated by heavy, spicy foods, especially if taken too hot or too cold.

A light and if possible liquid or semi-liquid diet should be resorted to for a while, or a fast started for a few days. Only food that is known to agree with the patient should be given, and it should be free from spices and other substances that would irritate the stomach. Overloading must be avoided by all means, even if the appetite is good. Pure water or, still better, flax seed tea, with the possible addition of mild fruit juices (e.g. apple), should be the only drinks allowed. To act healingly on the irritated lining and the ulcer, a tablespoonful of a mixture of pure olive oil with an equal amount of high-quality extract of malt should be given on an empty stomach, about an hour before meals. The bowels should be kept well regulated.

By proper treatment and strict adherence to a proper diet, the chances for recovery are good: The ulcer will gradually heal and will remain healed if the mistakes in diet that brought on the trouble are avoided. In extreme weakness, however, it is not advisable to resort to self-medication. Similarly, when bleeding is present, medical attention should be sought to rule out the possibility of cancer.

As an adjuvant in the treatment of ulcers of the stomach, there are a number of herbs that have proven to be of great merit. No. 94 is composed of herbs carefully selected and in their proper proportions.

Remedies: Use No. 94 or 95.

Assisting the Treatment: If constipated, use No. 26 or 27; but if bilious, then No. 6 should be used instead. In blood deficiency, use No. 11.

Stones or Gravel in Kidneys or Bladder

This trouble is caused by the collection of insoluble calcium-containing precipitates forming gravel or stones of various sizes in kidneys and bladder. If the deposits have formed in the kidneys, the pain extends from the mid-low back down to the bladder, rectum, and in men, the testicles, or, for women, the ovaries, and is more severely felt in the urinary passages. When these passages become obstructed by passing stones or gravel, scratching of the ureter may cause considerable pain and bleeding at times. If stones or gravel have formed in the bladder, the pain is felt at the neck of the bladder, extending downward to the end of the penis, especially as the last of the urine is voided. When the stone lodges over the mouth of the bladder, the flow of urine may at times be interrupted, or it may stop altogether, but a change in position may remove the obstruction and produce a normal flow again.

A number of herbs possess antilithic (anti-stone) and diuretic properties, which when properly combined and taken over a period of time have been found very helpful in loosening up and clearing the calcareous deposits. This combination of herbs will be found in No. 96.

Remedy: Use No. 96.

Assisting the Treatment: Hot sitz baths can be helpful. If constipated, use No. 26 or 27 in addition to the above.

Stones in Gallbladder
See GALLBLADDER, INFLAMMATION OF.

Stools
See "Symptoms," p. 24.

Stye
See EYES.

Sunburn
Remedy: No. 89.

Suppressed Menstruation
See MENSTRUATION, SUPPRESSED.

Sweating, Abnormal
See "Symptoms," p. 26.

Sweating Feet
See FEET, SWEATING.

Sweating, Offensive
See BODY ODOR.

Sweat-Producing Tea
See Nos. 21 and 22.

Swelling
See "Symptoms," p. 26.

Tapeworm

Several species of tapeworm can inhabit the human body and develop in the intestines. Their form is tapelike and consists of numerous flat segments or joints, of which the head, which is provided with suckers, is the smallest and the thinnest part. The tail end is the broadest, and is at times thrown off and expelled through the stools.

Inordinate appetite, disturbed digestion with a feeling of nausea, and colicky pains in the abdomen generally indicate the presence of this unwelcome guest. Sometimes, however, no symptoms are present, and the discharge of pieces of the worm, which are found in the stools, is the only positive evidence of its existence. The parts are passed from time to time in connected links or in single joints.

A number of good remedies aid in expelling the worm in a few hours without producing any harmful effect upon the system. The ingredients of No. 97 have proven quite effective and quick in action. This remedy, however, should be made fresh and then filled in capsules when needed, on account of its volatile nature and peculiar taste; only in this way can the full value of its specific action be obtained.

Remedy: Use No. 97.

Taste, Bitter and Pasty

See BILIOUSNESS; STOMACH DISORDERS.

Tea or Coffee Substitute

See No. 71, or *maté* leaves.

Tetter

See ECZEMA.

Throat, Sore

See TONSILLITIS.

Thumb-sucking

Remedy: No. 7.

Tired Feeling
See "Symptoms," p. 25.

Tonic Tea
See No. 71.

Tonsillitis (Sore throat; quinsy)
Tonsillitis begins with pain in the throat and difficulty in swallowing, accompanied by general body ache and sometimes chills. The throat is swollen, red, and inflamed, and one or both tonsils are enlarged and covered with a thick white mucus. Sometimes the tonsils become ulcerated. Headache and fever are often present, the tongue is coated, and the urine is highly colored and scanty.

To relieve the inflammation, apply cold, wet compresses around the neck and cover with a dry one; change it when it becomes warm, and leave one on overnight.

A gargle and mouthwash should be used freely to remove the slimy accumulations and to keep the throat antiseptic and clean.

Remedy: Use No. 98.

Assisting the Treatment: If constipated, use No. 26 or 27; but in the event a cold and fever are present, then use No. 20 instead. If appearing in connection with rheumatism, use No. 83.

Ulcers of the Stomach
See STOMACH DISORDERS.

Urination, Scanty, Painful, or Cloudy
See BLADDER, INFLAMMATION OR CATARRH OF OF.

Vertigo (Dizziness)
See CONSTIPATION; BILIOUSNESS; STOMACH DISORDERS; BLOOD PRESSURE, HIGH.

Vomiting
See "Symptoms," p. 23; also BILIOUSNESS; STOMACH DISORDERS.

Warts

These growths can be removed without pain and danger by the application of No. 99.

Remedy: No. 99.

Weakness, Nervous

See NERVOUSNESS.

Remedy: Herb Tonic, No. 11.

Weakness, Sexual

See SEXUAL WEAKNESS.

Whitlow of the Finger (Felon)

An inflammation of the finger, generally situated at the root of the nail. It is very painful and attended with swelling, soreness, and in severe cases with throbbing. When it progresses to the formation of pus, a small white spot appears, which, when opened, discharges pus.

This is a very stubborn disease if not properly attended to, and its healing depends to a great extent on the condition of the blood. The advice given under IMPURE BLOOD should therefore be followed. The local treatment should consist of bathing the affected parts in a strong decoction of equal parts of chamomile flowers and plantain leaves for about fifteen minutes. The area should then be dried thoroughly and the affected fingertips dipped in a jar of softened Healing Balsam No. 89, for about 5 minutes. Care should be taken that the balsam is not too hot. The adhering balsam may be left on the fingers overnight, using old gloves to prevent soiling the bedsheets.

Exposure of the affected fingers to water—especially to soap, detergent, or alkaline water—should be avoided by all means, as the irritation caused by these interferes with the healing process. Therefore washing, dishwashing, and similar tasks that necessitate exposure of the affected parts to water should be discontinued until the affected parts have been thoroughly healed.

Remedy: Use No. 89.

Assisting the Treatment: In impure blood, use No. 54 or 55. In stomach disorders, use No. 90 or 92.

Whooping Cough

This is a highly contagious disease, generally a child's disease. The patient should be isolated.

The complaint begins with a moderate bronchitis, but soon the cough grows worse, especially at night. Gradually it develops into severe shocks of cough in rapid succession, followed by a deep inhalation, or whoop, and the expectoration of a small amount of tough, sticky mucus. The patient should be kept in a warm, well-ventilated room. The food should be light, and the bowels well regulated.

Remedy: Use No. 100.

Assisting the Treatment: If constipated, use No. 28. If nervous and restless, use No. 69, to be rubbed on the chest and throat.

Worms

Intestinal parasites affecting the human body. (See also TAPE-WORM.) Paleness, restlessness, picking of the nose, irregular appetite, bad breath, itching in the rectum are generally the indications of the presence of worms. The sleep may be disturbed, the patient rolling from one side to the other, and grinding the teeth. These symptoms, however, may not all be present.

Remedy: Use No. 102.

Assisting the Treatment: If constipated, use No. 28. In bodily weakness, use No. 11.

Wounds

Clean them thoroughly with a mild solution of water and table salt. Boiled water should be used in making this solution. Stop the bleeding by applying sterilized clean cotton, then dress with salve, No. 103. This ointment has very healing and soothing properties. It is very useful in the treatment of wounds and sores of all kinds, including cuts, burns, scalds, and so on, and should be on hand all the time.

3

Herbal Recipes

Key to Herbal Recipes

RECIPE NUMBER	(MAUSERT NUMBER)	DESCRIPTION
1	(1)	Intestinal Elimination Powder
2	(3)	Powder for Asthma
3	(6)	Asthma Inhalation Powder
4	(9)	Asthma Cigarettes
5	(12)	Tea for Bed Wetting
6	(14)	Liver Capsules
7	(18)	Fingertip Dip
8	(21)	For Kidneys and Bladder
9	(24)	For High Blood Pressure—No. 1
10	(27)	For High Blood Pressure—No. 2
11	(30)	Herb Tonic
12	(32)	Deodorizing Lotion
13	(34)	Drawing and Healing Plaster
14	(36)	For Bronchial Cough
15	(39)	For Bronchial Cough—In Powder Form

Herbal Recipes

RECIPE NUMBER	(MAUSERT NUMBER)	DESCRIPTION
16	(42)	Bunion Balsam
17	(45)	Salve for Bunions
18	(48)	For Menopause
19	(51)	Chilblain Balsam
20	(54)	Cold-Breaker Capsules
21	(57)	Diaphoretic or Sweat-Producing Tea— Strong
22	(58)	Diaphoretic or Sweat-Producing Tea— Mild
23	(60)	Penetrating Massage Cream
24	(63)	For Colic in Infants
25	(65)	System-Regulator Capsules
26	(69)	Laxative Herbs for Constipation— Strong
27	(72)	Laxative Herbs for Constipation— Mild
28	(75)	Laxative Herbs for Constipation— For Children
29	(78)	Corn Remover
30	(81)	Tea for Coughs
31	(84)	Dandruff Hair Wash
32	(87)	Scalp Massage Oil
33	(90)	For Diabetes
34	(93)	Tea for Diarrhea
35	(96)	Drops for Diarrhea
36	(98)	Tea for Dropsy
37	(102)	Capsules for Dropsy
38	(105)	Hydragogue Capsules
39	(108)	For Dysentery
40	(111)	Ear Oil
41	(114)	External Lotion for Skin Eruptions (Eczema Lotion)
42	(126)	Herbs for Enema or Internal Bath
43	(129)	For Epilepsy

Herbal Recipes

RECIPE NUMBER	(MAUSERT NUMBER)	DESCRIPTION
44	(132)	Eye Lotion
45	(138)	Foot Powder
46	(141)	Herbs for Footbath
47	(147)	Bile Capsules
48	(148)	Gallbladder Remedy
49	(153)	Urinary Antiseptic
50	(156)	Urinary Antiseptic Capsules
51	(159)	For Gout
52	(162)	Herb Vinegar for External Use
53	(165)	For Hoarseness
54	(168)	For Blood Purifying, No. 1—Mild
55	(171)	For Blood Purifying, No. 2—Strong
56	(174)	Scabies Ointment
57	(177)	Renal Tea for Kidney Irregularities
58	(180)	Herbs for Douche
59	(189)	For Measles
60	(192)	Female Regulator Tea No. 1
61	(195)	Female Regulator Tea No. 2
62	(198)	Female Regulator Tea No. 3
63	(201)	Herb Mixture for Moths
64	(204)	Oil for Catarrh
65	(207)	Catarrh Balsam
66	(210)	Nerve Restorative Tea No. 1
67	(213)	Nerve Restorative Tea No. 2
68	(216)	Nerve Restorative Capsules
69	(219)	Analgesic Balm
70	(222)	Smelling Salts
71	(225)	Herb Health Tea
72	(228)	Neuralgia Anodyne
73	(231)	For Neuritis
74	(234)	For Night Sweats
75	(237)	Herbs for Reducing
76	(240)	Capsules for Hemorrhoids
77	(243)	Rectal Wash for Hemorrhoids

Herbal Recipes

RECIPE NUMBER	(MAUSERT NUMBER)	DESCRIPTION
78	(246)	Hemorrhoid Cones
79	(249)	Tea for Pleurisy
80	(252)	For Poison Oak and Poison Ivy
81	(255)	Poultice Powder
82	(258)	Mustard Poultice
83	(261)	For Rheumatism
84	(264)	Liniment for Rheumatism
85	(270)	For Sleeplessness
86	(273)	Restorative Herb Powder
87	(276)	Dusting Powder
88	(279)	Herbs for Soothing Compresses
89	(282)	Healing Balsam
90	(285)	For Gastritis
91	(288)	Capsules for Gastritis
92	(291)	For Nervous Dyspepsia
93	(294)	Capsules for Nervous Dyspepsia
94	(297)	For Ulcers of the Stomach and Duodenum—No. 1
95	(300)	For Ulcers of the Stomach and Duodenum—No. 2
96	(303)	For Stones or Gravel in Kidneys or Bladder
97	(306)	For Tapeworm
98	(309)	For Gargle and Mouthwash
99	(312)	For Warts
100	(315)	Whooping Cough Syrup
101	(318)	Inhalation for Whooping Cough
102	(321)	Worm Expeller
103	(324)	Antiseptic Salve

Notes on the Herbal Recipes

All recipes in this book have been thoroughly tested in regard to their effectiveness and reliability.* They cover all points of information in the treatment of the different diseases and are based on the practical experience of a lifetime. It is, therefore, unnecessary to give numerous recipes for each ailment, making their selection difficult and leaving the results that are expected to guesswork.

While some recipes listed in Mausert's original text are no longer readily available commercially, due to FDA insistence, we have retained those thought to be useful. Some herbs known to have toxic properties, such as mandrake and pokeroot, are retained in these recipes because the toxic properties would be experienced only after *repeated* use, over a long period of time. However, an overdose of mandrake could be fatal, and may cause birth defects if taken by a pregnant woman. This is why I recommend extreme caution in the use of these remedies. All medicines have associated risks, and where the problem is sufficient to warrant treatment the reader is advised to calculate the risk and/or consult a physician before using any remedies. In such conditions as may require medical attention (see remarks in "Symptoms," pages 21–26 and "Diseases," pages 27–75), the reader is advised to weigh with his or her physician the relative benefits of herbal remedies and other possible forms of treatment.

The common names (English-language names) given for the plants herein are those most commonly used today in the herb trade. For Latin names, see the Materia Medica section, pages 183–296. The few unfamiliar ingredients can be found in specialty pharmacies.

The recipes in this section were all written by Otto Mausert in precise weight and liquid measures, as this is the only way to get uniform and correctly dosed preparations. The expected results depend to a great extent on this exactness. The measurements found

*Before using *any* recipe in this book you are strongly advised to read the Materia Medica section (pp. 183–296) and note particularly the "cautions" which follow "Dose," in selected cases.

in so many herbal formulas, such as tablespoonful, cupful, handful, are very inaccurate, because tablespoons, cups, and hands are not all the same size. But a weight, such as an ounce, is always the same, no matter what is weighed—lead or feathers. A tablespoon of an herb, if fine cut or powdered, will hold twice as much, or more, as a tablespoon of a coarser cut. Therefore a preparation made by such a measure is inaccurate; it will be different every time it is made and the results will naturally be uncertain.

For this reason, we have retained Mausert's original measures in the first column in each recipe, for the greatest possible accuracy. For the sake of convenience, however, we have also provided roughly equivalent household measures, where appropriate, in the second column. In the case of some recipes, the constituents are too potent for approximate measurement, and strict liquid and weight measures must be used. We therefore urge, despite the approximate measures provided, that the most accurate measures be followed for precise formulas.

The following table of weights and measures has been used to determine equivalent measures.

---

1 *minim* (liquid measure) = 1 drop
1 *grain* (weight) = .065 gram, or 65 mg.
1 *drachm* or *dram* = 60 grains for weight and 60 minims (drops) for liquid measure
1 *drachm* or *dram* = 1 teaspoon (tsp.)
1 *ounce* = 8 drachms for weight or liquid measure
1 *ounce* = 2 tablespoons (Tbsp.)
1 *pound* = 16 ounces for weight
1 *pint* = 16 ounces liquid measure; 2 cups
1 *quart* = 2 pints liquid measure

For exact instructions on how to prepare herbal recipes, refer to the Introduction.

Herbal Recipes

The following equipment will be needed for the preparation of these recipes in your home.

Kitchen Equipment Needed

Heat source (stove, hot plate)
Pyrex pot for boiling water (with cover)
Glass or ceramic pot with tight-fitting lid
   for steeping infusions
Pyrex measuring cup
Measuring spoons
Medicine dropper
Mortar and pestle (ceramic)

NO. 1

Intestinal Elimination Powder

		DRACHMS	APPROX. EQUIV.
1.	Buckthorn Bark	6	6 tsp.
	Regulates bowels in a mild way.		
2.	Senna Fruit	4	4 tsp.
	Cleanses and regulates the system.		
3.	Oregon Graperoot	2	2 tsp.
	Has a tonic effect.		
4.	Sarsaparilla Root	2	2 tsp.
	Cleans blood; aids elimination.		
5.	Water Mint Leaves	2	2 tsp.
	Stimulates alimentary-tract secretions.		
6.	Licorice	2	2 tsp.
	Tonic to the mucous membrane.		
7.	Anise Seed	2	2 tsp.
	Relieves gas and prevents its formation.		

Herbal Recipes

Mix well and divide into twenty doses, using finely powdered material.

Directions: Take one dose in water, or mixed with jelly, jam, or honey, before retiring. In stubborn cases of constipation, a dose in the morning may also be taken. This recipe is especially useful when a laxative is indicated to clean the intestines in a mild way.

NO. 2
Powder for Asthma

		DRACHMS	APPROX. EQUIV.
1.	Indian Turnip	2	2 tsp.
	Facilitates expectoration.		
2.	Ephedra Herb	2	2 tsp.
	Useful in bronchial catarrh and asthma.		
3.	Lobelia	1	1 tsp.
	Stimulates the respiratory tract; relieves spasms.		
4.	Nerve Root	2	2 tsp.
	Quiets the nerves and relieves irritation.		
5.	Soap Bark	3	3 tsp.
	Loosens phlegm from bronchial tubes.		
6.	Cinnamon Bark	2	2 tsp.
	Acts as a local stimulant; pleasant aromatic.		
7.	Licorice	4	4 tsp.
	Relieves irritation; facilitates expectoration.		
8.	Elecampane Root	4	4 tsp.
	Allays cough and catarrhal inflammation of air passages.		

Mix well and divide into 20 doses, using finely powdered material.

Directions: Divide one dose in three parts and take one part in the morning, one at noon, and one at night, either mixed with a little honey or stirred up in some water.

This combination of herbs is a valuable remedy in affections of the throat and lungs, where slimy accumulations obstruct the air passages and cause shortness of breath, wheezing, and dry, painful coughing. It aids to loosen the phlegm, facilitates expectoration, relieves spasms, and stimulates the respiratory center.

NO. 3
Asthma Inhalation Powder

NOTE: This powder is used by inhalation only; the powder is burned and only the smoke is inhaled.

		OUNCES	APPROX. EQUIV.
1.	Stramonium Leaves Quiets spasms.	3	6 Tbsp.
2.	Black Henbane Leaves Soothes and quiets the nervous system.	¼	½ Tbsp.
3.	Lobelia Quiets spasms; promotes expectoration.	¼	½ Tbsp.
4.	Belladonna Leaves Sedative; painkiller.	¼	½ Tbsp.
5.	Cascarilla Bark A tonic to the system.	¼	½ Tbsp.
6.	Potassium Nitrate Promotes oxidation of plant material.	1	2 Tbsp.

Mix well and keep in a dry place, using powdered material.

Directions: Place about half a teaspoonful of the mixture on a piece of tin or porcelain, light it with a match, and inhale the fumes through the nostrils. This should be done immediately upon sensing the approach of an asthmatic paroxysm.

Caution: Do not take the powder internally.

NO. 4
Asthma Cigarettes

	OUNCES	APPROX. EQUIV.
1. Stramonium Leaves	3¼	6½ Tbsp.
Quiets spasms.		
2. Black Henbane Leaves	¼	½ Tbsp.
Soothes and quiets the nervous system.		
3. Belladonna Leaves	¼	½ Tbsp.
Sedative and painkiller.		
4. Potassium Nitrate	¼	½ Tbsp.
Promotes oxidation of plant material.		

Dissolve the potassium nitrate in one ounce of water; saturate the herbs, which have been previously well mixed, with the solution. Dry in moderate heat and roll or fill into cigarette papers.

Directions: These cigarettes are smoked and inhaled to relieve asthmatic paroxysms and other bronchial irritations.

NO. 5
Tea for Bed Wetting

	DRACHMS	APPROX. EQUIV.
1. Uva Ursi	6	6 tsp.
Gives tone to the urinary organs.		

2. St. John's wort	6	6 tsp.
Useful in urinary affections, especially when of a nervous nature.		
3. Yellow Ladies' Slipper Root	2½	2½ tsp.
Very quieting to the nervous system.		
4. Water Plantain	3	3 tsp.
A good urinary antiseptic and astringent.		
5. Belladonna Leaves	½	½ tsp.
Valuable to control involuntary muscular relaxation.		
6. Scouring Rush	2	2 tsp.
Strengthens the bladder.		

Mix well and divide into twenty doses, using herbs specially cut for tea purposes.

Directions: Add one dose to a cup of boiling water, let it stand for about 5 minutes, then strain. Give half of the infusion in the morning and the other half after supper, sweetened with honey if desired.

NO. 6
Liver Capsules

	GRAINS
1. Fringe Tree Extract	40
Relieves congestion of the liver.	
2. Wahoo Bark Extract	10
Stimulates the action of the liver.	
3. Mandrake Root Extract	4
Increases the flow of bile.	
4. Culver's Root Extract	20
Activates the liver.	
5. Poke Root Extract	10
Acts favorably on the glandular system.	

6. Aloe		60
Increases peristalsis; produces copious stools.		
7. Rhubarb		50
Increases muscular action of the intestines.		
8. Scullcap		2
Stimulates the nervous system.		

Mix thoroughly, using finely powdered material, and then pass through a small meshed sieve. Divide into 40 equal doses and fill capsules.

Directions: Two capsules once or twice a day, according to the laxative action required.

This recipe is especially useful in biliousness, sluggish liver, constipation of long standing, and catarrh of the stomach, bowels, or gallbladder. It will be found beneficial in dizziness, sick headache, nausea, and gassy conditions of stomach and bowels.

NO. 7
Fingertip Dip

		DRACHMS	APPROX. EQUIV.
1.	Quassia	8	8 tsp.
2.	Mugwort	4	4 tsp.
3.	Slippery Elm Bark	2	2 tsp.
4.	White Bryony	1	1 tsp.
5.	Grains of Paradise Seed	1	1 tsp.
	(All these herbs are selected for their unpleasant flavor.)		
6.	Sodium Benzoate	⅛	⅛ tsp.

Boil the herbs (nos. 1–5) with one pint of water down to half a pint, strain, and add no. 6, which acts as a preservative.

Directions: Moisten the fingertips with the liquid, allowing it to dry on. Repeat when washed off.

This preparation applied to fingertips is very effective in the prevention of nail biting and thumb and finger sucking. It acts as a reminder, is absolutely harmless, and should be tried by all those who have acquired any of these nasty habits.

NO. 8
For Kidneys and Bladder

		DRACHMS	APPROX. EQUIV.
1.	Uva Ursi	8	8 tsp.
	Very efficacious in catarrhal conditions of bladder.		
2.	Black Birch	2	2 tsp.
	A mild stimulant and astringent.		
3.	Couch Grass	8	8 tsp.
	Relieves irritation; acts to sooth and heal.		
4.	Buchu Leaves	4	4 tsp.
	Urinary antiseptic; relieves inflammation.		
5.	Juniper Berries	2	2 tsp.
	Stimulates the action of the genito-urinary tract.		
6.	Pipsissewa	3	3 tsp.
	A reliable diuretic.		
7.	Scouring Rush	3	3 tsp.
	Healing and soothing to the mucous membrane.		
8.	Celery Seed	2	2 tsp.
	Relieves the tendency to spasms.		

Mix well and divide into 20 doses, using herbs either especially cut for tea or in the powdered form.

Directions for Tea: Add one dose to 3 cups of boiling water, cover, boil slowly for about 2 or 3 minutes, let it stand for 10 minutes, then strain and take one third morning, noon, and night, either before or after meals. If boiling water is not available, use hot water and allow to stand for half an hour. It may be sweetened with honey, rock candy, sugar, etc., to suit taste.

Directions for Powder: Divide one dose in three parts, taking one third morning, noon, and night, either before or after meals. It may be taken in water or mixed with honey, jelly, or jam.

Whenever a reliable remedy is needed to relieve an inflamed catarrhal condition of the bladder, with its annoying symptoms of scanty or painful urination, thick cloudy urine, spasms in the bladder, constant desire to urinate, this recipe can be used to good advantage. It stimulates the action of the genito-urinary tract, relieves irritation, and tends to act as a soothing and healing agent to the mucous membrane of kidneys and bladder.

NO. 9
For High Blood Pressure
No. 1

		DRACHMS	APPROX. EQUIV.
1.	Rue Herb	1	1 tsp.
	Stimulates the nerves.		
2.	Golden Rod, European	1	1 tsp.
	Diuretic; relieves congestion.		
3.	Valerian Root	3	3 tsp.
	Quiets and soothes the nervous system.		
4.	Licorice	3	3 tsp.
	Acts mildly on the bowels.		

5.	Buckthorn	6	6 tsp.
	Cleanses the blood; stimulates stomach and bowels.		
6.	Speedwell	4	4 tsp.
	Stimulates the digestive functions.		
7.	Linden Flowers	2	2 tsp.
	Gentle stimulant and tonic.		

Mix well and divide into 20 doses, using the herbs especially cut for tea or in the powdered form.

Directions for Tea: Add one dose to 3 cups of boiling water, cover, boil slowly for about 2 or 3 minutes, let it stand for 10 minutes, then strain and take one third morning, noon, and night either before or after meals. If boiling water is not available, use hot water, and allow to stand for half an hour. It may be sweetened with honey, rock candy, sugar, etc., to suit taste.

Directions for Powder: Divide one dose in three parts, taking one third morning, noon, and night, either before or after meals. It may be taken in water or mixed with honey, jelly, or jam.

For those suffering from constipation, the following recipe, No. 10, is more appropriate.

NO. 10
For High Blood Pressure
No. 2

		DRACHMS	APPROX. EQUIV.
1.	Sassafras Bark	1½	1½ tsp.
	Valued for its blood-cleansing properties.		
2.	Golden Rod, European	1½	1½ tsp.
	Relieves congestion; diuretic.		
3.	Buckbean	1½	1½ tsp.
	Stimulates the system.		

4.	Black Cohosh Root Relieves nervous tension; reduces arterial action.	1½	1½ tsp.
5.	Poke Berry Stimulates glandular action.	1½	1½ tsp.
6.	Senna Fruit Activates the bowels.	6	6 tsp.
7.	Buckthorn Bark Cleanses and regulates the system.	15	15 tsp.
8.	Cassia Bark Stimulates the circulatory system.	1½	1½ tsp.

Mix well and divide into 20 doses, using the herbs either especially cut for tea or in the powdered form.

Directions for Tea: Add one dose to 3 cups of boiling water, cover, boil slowly for about 2 to 3 minutes, let it stand for 10 minutes, then strain and take one third morning, noon, and night, either before or after meals. If boiling water is not available, use hot water and allow to stand for half an hour. It may be sweetened with honey, rock candy, sugar, etc., to suit taste.

Directions for Powder: Divide one dose in three parts, taking one third morning, noon, and night, either before or after meals. It may be taken in water or mixed with honey, jelly, or jam.

These two recipes (nos. 9 and 10) are also highly valued in hardening of the arteries, fullness in the head, and in ear and head noises resulting from these troubles. If these noises are especially felt at night in bed, they are generally due to nervous disturbances or anemia and should be treated by removing the underlying cause.

NO. 11
Herb Tonic

		DRACHMS	APPROX. EQUIV.
1.	Cola Beans	¾	¾ tsp.
	Stimulates the appetite.		
2.	Senna	16	16 tsp.
	Cleanses the stomach and bowels.		
3.	Bitter Orange Peel	2½	2½ tsp.
	Aids in the digestion and assimilation of food.		
4.	Cinchona Bark	3	3 tsp.
	Invigorates the nervous system; aids digestion.		
5.	Yellow Gentian Root	4	4 tsp.
	A splendid digestive; useful in debility and exhaustion.		
6.	Cassia Bark	1	1 tsp.
	Tones up the circulatory system.		
7.	Coriander Seed	1	1 tsp.
	Relieves gas.		
8.	Cloves	¼	¼ tsp.
	Excites languid digestion; aromatic stimulant.		
		DROP	
9.	Oil of Orange	1	1 drop
	Improves taste of preparation.		
		QUART	
10.	Medicinal Muscatel Wine	1	1 quart
	In small single doses acts as a system tonic.		
		OUNCES	
11.	Sugar	4	8 Tbsp.
	Improves taste.		

Herbal Recipes

Extract herbs listed from no. 1 to 8 inclusive in the wine for 3 or 4 days, then press off the liquid and add nos. 9 and 11.

Directions: One tablespoonful three times a day. If appetite is poor, take before meals; otherwise, after meals.

Whenever a good blood and body builder is required, this recipe can be highly recommended. It builds and tones up the system, imparts strength and vitality to the weakened organs, and enriches the blood with needed vitamins and minerals. Excellent in general weakness, rundown condition, and exhaustion of the body and nervous system; also in low blood pressure, poor circulation, and anemia.

NO. 12
Deodorizing Lotion

		DRACHMS	APPROX. EQUIV.
1.	Soap Bark	1	1 tsp.
	Makes a soapy lather.		
2.	Red Oak Bark	2	2 tsp.
	Astringent.		
3.	Aluminum Chloride	1	1 tsp.
	Reduces perspiration.		
		GRAINS	
4.	Menthol	½	½ drop
	Antibacterial.		
		DROP	
5.	Oil of Rhodium	1	1 drop
	Scent.		
		OUNCES	
6.	Distilled Water	4	8 Tbsp.

Boil items no. 1 and no. 2 in no. 6 slowly for about 5 minutes, let stand until lukewarm, then strain and add nos. 3, 4, and 5. Shake until no. 4 is dissolved. Add sufficient distilled water to make four ounces.

Directions: Apply to affected parts every other night and let it dry. Wash the applied part the next morning with water.

A very useful preparation to overcome body odor and offensive perspiration quickly and effectively.

NO. 13
Drawing and Healing Plaster

		DRACHMS	APPROX. EQUIV.
1.	Camphorated Brown Plaster	7	7 tsp.
	Protects inflamed skin and subcutaneous tissue.		
2.	Navy Pitch	1½	1½ tsp.
	Promotes eruption.		
3.	Lamb's Fat	½	½ tsp.
	Holds ingredients together.		
4.	Cottonseed Oil	7	7 tsp.
	Emollient.		

Melt nos. 1, 2, 3; when half cooled, add no. 4 and mix.

Directions: Spread on a clean piece of linen as thick as the blade of a knife and big enough to cover the boil or inflamed pimple. Hold in place by adhesive tape and renew morning and night. When the discharge of pus ceases, in order to complete the healing of the wound, apply Antiseptic Salve, no. 103.

NO. 14
For Bronchial Cough

		DRACHMS	APPROX. EQUIV.
1.	Yerba Santa	2½	2½ tsp.
	Stimulates the respiratory organs.		
2.	Wild Cherry Bark	4	4 tsp.
	Allays irritation and aids expectoration.		
3.	Irish Moss	2	2 tsp.
	Very useful in chronic pectoral affections.		
4.	Licorice	9	9 tsp.
	Facilitates expectoration.		
5.	Comfrey	2	2 tsp.
	Relieves congestion in chest and bronchial tubes.		
6.	Elecampane Root	6	6 tsp.
	Very helpful in chronic pulmonary affections.		
7.	Lobelia	½	½ tsp.
	Relaxes the system; stimulates the respiratory center.		
8.	Anise Seed	2	2 tsp.
	An aromatic expectorant of value.		

Mix well and divide into 20 doses, using herbs especially cut for tea.

Directions: Add one dose to 3 cups of boiling water, cover, boil slowly for about 2 to 3 minutes, let stand for 10 minutes, then strain and take one third morning, noon, and night, either before or after meals. If boiling water is not available, use hot water and allow to stand for half an hour. It may be sweetened with honey, rock candy, sugar, etc., to suit taste.

NO. 15
For Bronchial Cough
In Powder Form

		DRACHMS	APPROX. EQUIV.
1.	Squill	1	1 tsp.
	An excellent expectorant and stimulant for the bronchial tubes.		
2.	Ipecac Root	½	½ tsp.
	Loosens phlegm and relieves bronchial irritation.		
3.	Lobelia Herb	1½	1½ tsp.
	Stimulates the respiratory organs.		
4.	Irish Moss	6	6 tsp.
	Relieves irritation; soothes and heals.		
5.	Soap Bark	4	4 tsp.
	Facilitates expectoration.		
6.	Fennel	8	8 tsp.
	An aromatic expectorant.		

Mix well and divide into 20 doses, using finely powdered material.

Directions: Divide one dose in three parts, taking one third morning, noon, and night, either before or after meals. It may be taken in water or mixed with honey, jelly, or jam.

The foregoing two recipes (nos. 14 and 15) will be found especially valuable in coughs and colds affecting the bronchial tubes and lungs. Dry and painful coughing with soreness and hoarseness of the throat will be greatly benefited by the soothing and healing effect of these herbs. They tend to relieve irritation and congestion in chest and air passages, facilitate expectoration, and stimulate the respiratory organs.

Herbal Recipes

NO. 16
Bunion Balsam

	GRAINS	APPROX. EQUIV.
1. Balsam, Peru Promotes healing.	15	¼ tsp.
2. Aloe Powder Soothing; promotes healing.	15	¼ tsp.
3. Myrrh Powder Astringent; healing.	25	5/12 tsp. (a little less than ½ tsp.)
4. Benzoin Powder Antiseptic.	60	1 tsp.
5. Iodine Powder Antiseptic.	15	¼ tsp.
6. Menthol Antibacterial.	15	¼ tsp.
	OUNCES	
7. Flexible Collodion Forms protective film.	1	2 Tbsp.

Mix well in a bottle, let stand for a few days, occasionally shaking the mixture, then strain off the clear liquid, discarding the sediment.

Directions: Apply to bunions with a brush morning and night.

This recipe is a well-tried and very effective preparation for bunions and inflamed joints.

NO. 17
Salve for Bunions

		GRAINS	APPROX. EQUIV.
1.	Phenol	20	⅓ tsp.
	Antiseptic; anesthetic.		
2.	Menthol	20	⅓ tsp.
	Antibacterial.		
3.	Camphor	20	⅓ tsp.
	Antiseptic; promotes circulation to affected part.		
		DRACHMS	
4.	Lanolin	3	3 tsp.
	Ointment base; protects against moisture.		
5.	Bay Tree Oil	3	3 tsp.
	Astringent.		
6.	Cottonseed Oil	8	8 tsp.
	Stimulates healing.		
7.	Belladonna Extract	½	½ tsp.
	Relieves pain.		
		DROPS	
8.	Oil of Cloves	10	10 drops

Make into a smooth salve.

Direction: Apply to bunions morning and night. This salve should be used when the skin is open. Calluses on bunions can be removed with No. 29.

Herbal Recipes

NO. 18
For Menopause

		DRACHMS	APPROX. EQUIV.
1.	White Poplar Bark	3	3 tsp.
	Uterine and general tonic.		
2.	Partridge Berry Herb	2	2 tsp.
	A great Indian remedy for female ir-regularities.		
3.	Beth Root	3	3 tsp.
	Uterine tonic.		
4.	Cramp Bark	3	3 tsp.
	Relieves menstrual pain and cramps.		
5.	Button Snakeroot	2	2 tsp.
	Uterine tonic.		
6.	Damiana Leaves	4	4 tsp.
	Increases the power of the reproductive organs.		
7.	Cassia Bark	3	3 tsp.
	Tones the circulatory system; arrests hemorrhages.		

Mix well and divide into 20 doses, using the herbs either especially cut for tea or in the powdered form.

Directions for Tea: Add one dose to 3 cups of boiling water, cover, boil slowly for about 2 to 3 minutes, let stand for 10 minutes, then strain and take one third morning, noon, and night, either before or after meals. If boiling water is not available, use hot water and allow to stand for half an hour. It may be sweetened with honey, rock candy, etc., to suit taste.

Directions for Powder: Divide one dose in three parts, taking one third morning, noon, and night, either before or after meals. It may be taken in water, or mixed with honey, jelly, or jam.

This combination of herbs has proven very useful and efficient in menopause and its accompanying symptoms known as hot flushes, in dizziness, headaches, nervous irritability, pain in loins and back, and in general weakness.

NO. 19
Chilblain Balsam

		DROPS
1.	Oil of Mustard Stimulates circulation to affected part.	4
2.	Oil of Eucalyptus Antiseptic.	20

		GRAINS
3.	Menthol Reduces pain sensation.	10

		DRACHMS
4.	Tincture of Iodine Counterirritant.	2
5.	Flexible Collodion Forms protective film.	6

Place in bottle and mix well; allow to stand for a few hours.

Directions: Apply with brush to affected parts before retiring; if the skin is broken use Salve for Bunions, No. 17. These recipes are serviceable and effective.

NO. 20
Cold Breaker Capsules

		GRAINS
1.	Aconite Root Reduces fever; relieves pain.	5

2.	Ginger	5
	Stimulates the nervous system.	
3.	Gum Camphor	5
	Incites circulation; stimulates heart action.	
4.	Aloin	5
	A derivative of aloe; regulates and cleanses the digestive tract.	
5.	Yellow Jessamine	2
	Useful in fever, ague, influenza.	
6.	Turmeric Root	2
	Stimulant aromatic.	
7.	Mandrake Extract	5
	Acts on liver and bowels.	
8.	Quinine	50
	Breaks fever and chills.	
		DROP
9.	Oil of Anise	1
	Aromatic.	

Mix thoroughly, using finely powdered material, and then pass through a small-meshed sieve. Divide into 20 equal parts and fill capsules.

Directions: Take one capsule morning, noon, and night; if bowels move too freely, take only one capsule in the morning and one at night.

These capsules have proven to be very effective in the different forms of colds, chills, fever, and catarrhal conditions due to colds.

NO. 21
Diaphoretic or Sweat-Producing Tea—Strong

		DRACHMS	APPROX. EQUIV.
1.	Elder Flowers Promotes fluid secretions.	1½	1½ tsp.
2.	Linden Flowers A gentle stimulant and diaphoretic.	1½	1½ tsp.
3.	Pennyroyal Stimulates secretions and opens the pores.	1½	1½ tsp.
4.	Boneset Produces sweating; valuable tonic in fevers.	1½	1½ tsp.
5.	Jaborandi Leaves Produces profuse perspiration.	4	4 tsp.

Mix well and divide into 5 doses, using herbs especially cut for tea.
Directions: Add one dose to 2 cups of boiling water, let stand for about 3 to 5 minutes, then strain and drink before going to bed.

This recipe is an excellent one to produce sweating, which is so helpful as an adjunct in the treatment of colds, influenza, ague, malaria, and all feverish conditions. For children or for a mild diaphoretic, No. 22 should be used.

NO. 22
Diaphoretic or Sweat-Producing Tea—Mild

		DRACHMS	APPROX. EQUIV.
1.	Boneset A reliable diaphoretic.	2	2 tsp.

2.	Elder Flowers	4	4 tsp.
	Promotes perspiration.		
3.	Black Birch Leaves	2	2 tsp.
	Acts on kidneys and opens the pores.		
4.	Water Mint Leaves	2	2 tsp.
	Aromatic stimulant.		

Mix well and divide into 10 doses, using herbs especially cut for tea.

Directions: Add one dose to 2 cups of boiling water, let stand for about 3 to 5 minutes, then strain and drink hot before going to bed. For children the amount of water may be decreased and the tea may be sweetened.

NO. 23
Penetrating Massage Cream

		GRAINS	APPROX. EQUIV.
1.	Gum Camphor	45	¾ tsp.
	Antiseptic; stimulates circulation.		
2.	Menthol	30	½ tsp.
	Produces cooling sensation; counterirritant.		
		DROPS	
3.	Oil of Wintergreen	75	1¼ tsp.
	Counterirritant.		
4.	Oil of Black Mustard	8	8 drops
	Stimulates circulation.		
5.	Oil of Geranium	15	15 drops
	Imparts sweet scent.		
		DRACHMS	
6.	Sesame Oil	5	5 tsp.
	Softens skin.		

7.	Lanolin	10	10 tsp.
	Cream base.		
8.	White Petrolatum	2½	2½ tsp.
	Ointment base.		
9.	Rose Water	6	6 tsp.
	Sweet scent.		

Melt nos. 6 and 7; when half cooled, add nos. 1, 2, 3, 4, and 5. Stir until dissolved, then add no. 9, previously warmed a little, and keep stirring until a smooth cream is obtained.

Directions: Rub well into affected parts morning and night.

This cream will be found to be an excellent massage cream for use in poor circulation, coldness, numbness, etc.

NO. 24
For Colic in Infants

		DRACHMS	APPROX. EQUIV.
1.	Fennel Seed	4	4 tsp.
	Relieves pain from gas pressure.		
2.	Water Mint Leaves	3	3 tsp.
	Relieves cramps and pain.		
3.	Valerian	1	1 tsp.
	Quiets and soothes stomach and bowels.		
4.	Chamomile Flowers	2	2 tsp.
	Removes gases; relieves spasms and colicky pains.		

Mix well and divide into 20 doses, using herbs especially cut for tea.

Directions: Add one dose to 1½ cups of boiling water, let it steep for about 5 minutes, then strain and give in 5 or 6 doses during the day, preferably warm in milk or plain.

This harmless but effective herb combination has a quieting and soothing effect, relieves gases and the pains and spasms caused by them. It should be on hand at all times.

NO. 25
System Regulator Capsules

	GRAINS
1. Mandrake Root Extract Incites the liver to healthy action.	8
2. Ginger Root, powdered Acaminative.	48
3. Wahoo Bark Extract A great Indian remedy to stimulate liver and bowels.	48
4. Cayenne Pepper Stimulates lower bowel.	24
5. Aloe Powder Increases bowel activity, promotes copi- ous stools.	96
	DROPS
6. Oil of Caraway Seeds Relieves gas and spasmodic pains.	6

Mix thoroughly, then pass through a small-meshed sieve. Divide into 48 equal doses and fill capsules.

Directions: One or two capsules before retiring, as needed. Whenever a general cleansing of the whole system and proper regulation of stomach, liver, and bowels are needed, this recipe will give satisfactory results. Its action is mild, harmless, and safe.

NO. 26

Laxative Herbs for Constipation—Strong

		DRACHMS	APPROX. EQUIV.
1.	Yellow Dock Root	2	2 tsp.
	Stimulates the bowels.		
2.	Violet Leaves	2	2 tsp.
	Has a tonic laxative effect.		
3.	Senna Fruit	4	4 tsp.
	Increases muscular action of stomach and bowels.		
4.	Culver's Root	3	3 tsp.
	A great stimulant for liver and bowels.		
5.	Water Mint	1	1 tsp.
	Relieves gas.		
6.	Oregon Grape Root	2	2 tsp.
	Causes easy bowel movements; aids digestion.		
7.	Licorice	4	4 tsp.
	Mild laxative.		
8.	Mandrake Root	2	2 tsp.
	Incites liver action; increases flow of bile.		

Mix well and divide into 20 doses, using herbs either especially cut for tea or in the powdered form.

Directions for Tea: Add one dose to 1 or 2 cups of boiling water. Boil for 2 or 3 minutes, let stand it for about 10 minutes, then strain and drink before retiring. If boiling water is not available, use hot water and allow to stand for half an hour.

Directions for Powder: Take one dose, either in water or mixed with honey, jelly, or jam, before retiring.

NO. 27
Laxative Herbs for Constipation—Mild

		DRACHMS	APPROX. EQUIV.
1.	Wild Thyme	1	1 tsp.
	Useful in debility of stomach and bowels.		
2.	Buckthorn Bark	6	6 tsp.
	A valuable laxative, especially in habitual constipation.		
3.	Sassafras Bark	2	2 tsp.
	Tones the bowels and cleanses the blood.		
4.	Oregon Grape Root	2	2 tsp.
	Acts mildly on liver and bowels.		
5.	Knot Grass	3	3 tsp.
	Soothes and heals the mucous lining of bowels.		
6.	Licorice Root	2	2 tsp.
	Has a mild action on the bowels.		
7.	Senna Fruit	4	4 tsp.
	Stimulates the action of the bowels.		

Mix well and divide into 20 doses, using herbs either especially cut for tea or in powdered form.

Directions for Tea: Add one dose to 1 or 2 cups of boiling water, boil for 2 or 3 minutes, let it stand for about 10 minutes, then strain and drink before retiring. If boiling water is not available, use hot water and allow to stand for half an hour.

Directions for Powder: Take one dose, either in water or mixed with honey, jelly, or jam, before retiring.

Nos. 26 and 27 are good formulas for constipation and consequently are excellent for the treatment of diseases arising from disorders of the stomach, liver, and bowels. They promote a healthy secretion of the gastric and digestive juices, which aid in performing the functions of the inner organs. They are therefore invaluable in cases of constipation, biliousness, coated tongue, foul breath, and so on, caused by lazy action of the liver and sluggish bowels. Where a stronger action is indicated, No. 26 should be used. No. 27, on the other hand, is mild in its action.

NO. 28
Laxative Herbs for Constipation in Children

		DRACHMS	APPROX. EQUIV.
1.	Licorice Root	6	6 tsp.
	Mild tonic laxative.		
2.	Pansy Herb	2	2 tsp.
	Stimulates secretion; cleans blood.		
3.	Crimson Clover Blossoms	2	2 tsp.
	Cleanses and regulates the system.		
4.	Senna Fruit	2	2 tsp.
	Stimulates the action of stomach and bowels.		
5.	Fennel Seed	4	4 tsp.
	Relieves gas, colic, and griping pains.		
6.	Buckthorn	4	4 tsp.
	Regulates and cleans the bowels in a mild way.		

Mix well and divide into 20 doses, using herbs either especially cut for tea or in the powdered form.

Directions: For tea and powder, prepare the same as No. 27, except use one cup of boiling water instead of two. Dose may be reduced or increased according to constitution and age of the child.

In children, with their undeveloped, tender organs, special care must be taken not to use harsh and drastic laxatives to overcome constipation. In No. 28, the mild and harmless herbs have been so combined as to give best results.

NO. 29
Corn Remover

		DROPS	APPROX. EQUIV.
1.	Castor Oil	15	¼ tsp.
	Oil base.		
		GRAINS	
2.	Salicylic Acid	15	¼ tsp.
	Softens horny skin.		
		DRACHMS	
3.	Collodion	2	2 tsp.
	Forms protective film.		
4.	Spirits of Ether	½	2 tsp.
	Solvent.		
		DROPS	
5.	Alkanet Root Extract: 1-in-10 solution	2	2 drops
	Coloring agent; astringent.		

Dissolve no. 2 in nos. 3 and 4, then add nos. 1 and 5.

Directions: Apply with brush to corns and calluses morning and night until skin becomes white under the coating, then soak the foot in warm water and remove the hardened skin with fingernail. Repeat if necessary.

This recipe is safe and reliable for the removal of corns, calluses, hardened skin of any kind, and warts, without pain or discomfort.

NO. 30
Tea for Coughs

		DRACHMS	APPROX. EQUIV.
1.	Thyme Leaves	4	4 tsp.
	Quieting and soothing to the mucous membrane.		
2.	Soap Bark	2	2 tsp.
	Aids expectoration.		
3.	Couch Grass	6	6 tsp.
	Loosens mucous accumulations.		
4.	Lobelia Herb	½	½ tsp.
	Stimulates the respiratory centers.		
5.	Lungwort Herb	5	5 tsp.
	A valuable expectorant.		
6.	Irish Moss	2	2 tsp.
	Very useful in chronic pectoral affections.		
7.	Elecampane Root	5½	5½ tsp.
	Facilitates expectoration.		
8.	Licorice	9	9 tsp.
	Relieves irritation; loosens phlegm.		
9.	Anise Seed	6	6 tsp.
	Allays irritation in the air passages.		

Mix well and divide into 20 doses, using herbs especially cut for tea.

Directions: Add one dose to 3 cups boiling water, cover, boil slowly for about 2 to 3 minutes, let it stand for 10 minutes, then strain and take one third morning, noon, and night before or after meals. If boiling water is not available, use hot water and allow to stand for half an hour. It may be sweetened with honey, rock candy, sugar, etc., to suit taste.

This is a very good recipe for the treatment of affections of the bronchial tubes and lungs. Coughs and colds settled in these organs, and tickling and irritation in the throat, are quickly relieved by its quieting and soothing effect. It also helps loosen phlegm and facilitates expectoration.

NO. 31
Dandruff Hair Wash

		DRACHMS	APPROX. EQUIV.
1.	Quassia Bark	2	2 tsp.
2.	Colocynth Pulp	1	1 tsp.
3.	Soap Bark	12	12 tsp.
	Forms lather.		
4.	Red Oak Bark	2	2 tsp.
	Astringent.		
5.	Black Walnut Leaves	1½	1½ tsp.
	Astringent.		
6.	Black Birch Leaves	1½	1½ tsp.
	Astringent.		

Mix well and divide into 20 doses, using herbs especially cut for tea.

Directions: Boil one dose in a pint of water slowly for about 5 minutes, then strain and use the liquid while still warm as a shampoo before retiring, washing and brushing the scalp thoroughly with the decoction. When nearly dry, massage the scalp well with No. 32, working it in well with the fingertips, moving the skin in a circular movement and then loosening the scalp by pulling the hair. Hair coming out by this procedure would fall out anyway. It is the new hair that will stay and be healthy and strong. Use the shampoo twice a week, but No. 32 daily.

NO. 32
Scalp Massage Oil

		OUNCES
1.	Castor Oil Oil base.	1
2.	Oil of Burdock Root (Klettenwurzel oil, German) Oil base.	2½
3.	Liquid Petrolatum Softens skin.	½

		DROPS
4.	Oil of English Lavender Scent.	15

		GRAINS
5.	Alkanet Root Extract Astringent; coloring agent.	½

Mix well and rub into scalp as directed under instructions for No. 31. Loss of hair is mostly due to an unhealthy condition of the scalp, brought on by parasitic life of either plant or animal origin, or to inactivity of the sebaceous glands and poor circulation. No. 31 and No. 32 will give good results in all these disturbances if the instructions are carefully followed. They tend to clean the scalp, help the circulation of the blood, invigorate the hair follicles, and keep the scalp in a sanitary condition. If used faithfully for a while, they will tend to stop the falling out of the hair and stimulate the growth of new hair. Very often the loss of hair is also due to nervous disturbances; in such cases the nervous system should be treated at the same time in order to get best results.

Herbal Recipes

NO. 33
For Diabetes

		DRACHMS	APPROX. EQUIV.
1.	Cleavers Herb Relieves inflammation of the urinary tract.	2	2 tsp.
2.	Couch Grass Heals and soothes.	4	4 tsp.
3.	Uva Ursi Gives tone to urinary organs; assists metabolism.	6	6 tsp.
4.	Spotted Wintergreen Improves bodily functions.	2	2 tsp.
5.	Jambul Berries Considered of exceptional merit in diabetes.	4	4 tsp.
6.	Whortleberry Leaves Used extensively in Europe in diabetes.	2	2 tsp.

Mix well and divide into 20 doses, using herbs either especially cut for tea or in the powdered form.

Directions for Tea: Add one dose to 3 cups of boiling water, cover, boil slowly for about 2 to 3 minutes, let it stand for 10 minutes, then strain and take one third morning, noon, and night, either before or after meals. If boiling water is not available, use hot water and allow to stand for half an hour. It may be sweetened by adding fruit juice.

Directions for Powder: Divide one dose in three parts, taking one third morning, noon, and night, either before or after meals. It should be taken with water.

NO. 34
Tea for Diarrhea

		DRACHMS	APPROX. EQUIV.
1.	Alum Root	4	4 tsp.
	Arrests excessive mucous discharges.		
2.	Colombo Root	4	4 tsp.
	Valuable in inflammatory diseases of stomach and bowels.		
3.	Ginger	3	3 tsp.
	Effective for loose bowels.		
4.	White Oak Bark	4	4 tsp.
	Relieves diarrhea and dysentery.		
5.	Pomegranate	8	8 tsp.
	Effective astringent, very useful in diarrhea.		
6.	Black Birch Leaves	4	4 tsp.
	Stimulates the mucous membranes of the bowels.		
7.	Wild Sage	3	3 tsp.
	Relieves inflammation.		

Mix well and divide into 20 doses, using herbs either especially cut for tea or in powdered form.

Directions for Tea: Add one dose to 3 cups of boiling water, cover, boil slowly for about 2 to 3 minutes, let it stand for 10 minutes, then strain and take one third morning, noon, and night, either before or after meals. If boiling water is not available, use hot water and allow to stand for half an hour. It may be sweetened with honey, rock candy, sugar, etc., to suit taste.

Directions for Powder: Divide one dose in three parts, taking one third morning, noon, and night, either before or after meals. It may be taken in water or mixed with honey, jelly, or jam.

NO. 35
Drops for Diarrhea

		DRACHMS	APPROX. EQUIV.
1.	Ginger Powder	1	1 tsp.
	Stimulates action of stomach and bowels.		
2.	Cayenne Pepper Powder	¼	¼ tsp.
	Increases the blood flow to affected parts.		
3.	Rhatany Root Powder	1½	1½ tsp.
	Has powerful astringent properties.		
4.	Yellow Ladies' Slipper Root	1½	1½ tsp.
	Quiets the affected nerves.		
5.	Tormentil Root	1½	1½ tsp.
	Useful astringent in diarrhea and dysentery.		
6.	Red Oak Bark Root	1½	1½ tsp.
	Stops mucous discharges; acts as an antiseptic.		
7.	Gum Camphor Powder	½	½ tsp.
	Refreshes and revives body functions.		
8.	Oil of Peppermint	½	½ tsp.
	Allays griping and spasms; aids digestion.		
9.	Tincture Valerian	22½	22½ tsp.
	Relieves spasms and cramps.		
10.	Ether	2½	2½ tsp.
	Relieves pain and spasms.		

Extract the powders with the liquids for 2 to 3 days, then strain and add no. 8.

Directions: Take 15 to 20 drops, three or four times a day, in warm water. These drops may be added to the infusion tea made in No. 34.

NO. 36
Tea for Dropsy

		DRACHMS	APPROX. EQUIV.
1.	Button Snakeroot	6	6 tsp.
	Stimulates the elimination of waste products.		
2.	Squill	1	1 tsp.
	Incites the flow of urine.		
3.	Black Indian Hemp Root	6	6 tsp.
	Removes dropsical accumulations.		
4.	Great Celandine Herb	6	6 tsp.
	Increases the flow of urine; effective hydragogue.		
5.	Foxglove Leaves	1	1 tsp.
	Stimulates heart action; helps the absorption of dropsical fluid accumulations.		

Mix well and divide into 20 doses, using herbs especially cut for tea.

Directions: Add one dose to 3 cups of boiling water (do not boil), let stand for about 10 minutes, then strain, and drink one third of the infusion morning, noon, and night.

For a recipe that acts similarly and is in a more convenient form, see No. 37, which is put up in capsules.

NO. 37
Capsules for Dropsy

		GRAINS	APPROX. EQUIV.
1.	Foxglove	30	½ tsp.
	Stimulates heart action; helps the absorption of dropsical fluid accumulations.		
2.	Squill	30	½ tsp.
	Incites the flow of urine.		
3.	Buchu Leaves Extract	30	½ tsp.
	A very useful diuretic and eliminator.		
4.	Uva Ursi Extract	60	1 tsp.
	Stimulates the urinary organs.		

Mix thoroughly, using finely powdered material. Divide into 30 equal doses and fill capsules.

Directions: One capsule morning, noon, and night with some warm water.

In order to help the elimination of water, not only through the kidneys but also through the bowels, No. 38, which is a hydragogue cathartic, should be used in connection with No. 36 or 37.

NO. 38
Hydragogue Capsules

		GRAINS
1.	Jalap Root Resin	5
	Produces copious, watery stools.	
2.	Gamboge Resin	12½
	An effective hydragogue cathartic.	
3.	Mandrake Root Resin	2½
	Incites liver and bowels to greater activity.	

4. Culver's Root Extract   10
   Causes watery evacuation of the bowels.
5. Henbane Extract   5
   Relieves irritation in the nervous system.
6. Aloe, Powdered   15
   Induces watery bowel movements.

Mix thoroughly. Divide into 20 equal doses and fill capsules.

Directions: Two capsules once a day. If watery stools are not obtained, the dose may be increased slightly.

NO. 39
For Dysentery

		DRACHMS	APPROX. EQUIV.
1.	Pomegranate Bark	11	11 tsp.
	Invigorates the weakened mucous lining of the bowels.		
2.	Tormentil Root	3	3 tsp.
	Strengthens the action of the bowels.		
3.	Galangal Root	3	3 tsp.
	Relieves catarrhal conditions.		
4.	Blackberry Bark	3	3 tsp.
	Known for its valuable astringent properties.		
5.	Shepherd's Purse Herb	3	3 tsp.
	Contracts blood vessels; stops bleeding.		
6.	Canada Fleabane Herb	3	3 tsp.
	Contracts loose tissues.		
7.	Alum Root	4	4 tsp.
	Arrests hemorrhages and mucous discharges.		

Mix well and divide into 20 doses, using herbs either especially cut for tea or in the powdered form.

Directions for Tea: Add one dose to 3 cups of boiling water, cover, boil slowly for about 2 to 3 minutes, let it stand for 10 minutes, then strain and take one third morning, noon, and night, either before or after meals. If boiling water is not available, use hot water and allow to stand for half an hour. It may be sweetened with honey, rock candy, sugar, etc., to suit taste.

Directions for Powder: Divide one dose in three parts, taking one third morning, noon, and night, either before or after meals. It may be taken in water or mixed with honey, jelly, or jam.

No. 35 should always be used in connection with No. 39 and may be taken right in the tea, or with the powder.

NO. 40
Ear Oil

		DROPS	APPROX. EQUIV.
1.	Oil of Cajeput Counterirritant.	8	8 drops
2.	Oil of Rue Soothing to the nerves.	8	8 drops
3.	Oil of Cloves Stimulant.	4	4 drops
		DRACHMS	
4.	Camphorated Oil Relieves pain.	4	4 tsp.
5.	Oil of Sesame Softening agent.	4	4 tsp.
		GRAIN	
6.	Alkanet Root Extract Astringent; coloring agent.	¼	¼ drop (tiny pinch)

Mix well.

Directions: Drop into the ear about 5 to 6 drops before retiring and in the morning.

This recipe is recommended to improve hardness of hearing, ringing and buzzing in the ear, and to soften and remove ear wax, which is often responsible for noises in the ear. Nervous and anemic people are often bothered with ear noises, especially at night in bed; in such instances, the underlying cause should receive attention.

NO. 41
External Lotion for Skin Eruptions (Eczema Lotion)

		DRACHMS
1.	Great Celandine	1
	A traditional home remedy for skin diseases.	
2.	Frostwort	1
	Astringent.	
		OUNCES
3.	Distilled Water	6
		GRAINS
4.	Salicylic Acid	2 (approx.)
	Removes horny skin; germicide; stimulant.	
		DRACHMS
5.	Resorcinol	2
	Anti-itching agent; antiseptic.	
6.	Glycerine	4
	Softens and moistens the skin.	

Boil nos. 1 and 2 slowly in 6 ounces of distilled water down to 4 ounces, strain, and add nos. 4, 5, and 6 in the decoction, then add sufficient distilled water to bring it up to 6 ounces.

Directions: Apply to affected parts two or three times a day.

NO. 42
Herbs for Enema or Internal Bath

		OUNCES	APPROX. EQUIV.
1.	Wild Sage	1½	1½ tsp.
	Relieves inflammation.		
2.	Soap Bark	1½	1½ tsp.
	Makes a lather.		
3.	Red Oak Bark	1½	1½ tsp.
	Contracts swollen tissues.		
4.	Plantain Leaves	1	1 tsp.
	Promotes healing.		
5.	Flax Seed	3	3 tsp.
	Soothing to the mucous membranes.		
6.	Rosemary Leaves	1½	1½ tsp.
	Soothes the nerves.		

Mix well and divide into 10 doses.

Directions: Add one dose to 2 quarts of boiling water, boil for about 3 minutes, allow to cool until lukewarm, then strain and use as an enema.

NO. 43
For Epilepsy

		DRACHMS	APPROX. EQUIV.
1.	Parnassia Herb	8	8 tsp.
	Highly valuable in epilepsy and convulsions.		

2.	Mugwort Herb	4	4 tsp.
	Beneficial in nervous irritability and in fits.		
3.	Peony Root	5	5 tsp.
	Relieves irritation of the nerve centers.		
4.	Valerian Root	6	6 tsp.
	Strengthens the nervous system.		
5.	Horse Nettle Berries	5	5 tsp.
	Very effective in epilepsy and convulsions.		
6.	Cassia Bark	2	2 tsp.
	Tones up the circulatory system.		

Mix well and divide into 20 doses, using herbs either especially cut for tea or in the powdered form.

Directions for Tea: Add one dose to 3 cups of boiling water, cover, boil slowly about 2 to 3 minutes, let it stand for 10 minutes, then strain and take one third morning, noon, and night, either before or after meals. If boiling water is not available, use hot water and allow it to stand for half an hour. It may be sweetened with honey, rock candy, sugar, etc., to suit taste.

Directions for Powder: Divide one dose in three parts, taking one third morning, noon, and night, either before or after meals. It may be taken in water or mixed with honey, jelly, or jam.

NO. 44
Eye Lotion

		GRAINS
1.	Eyebright Herb	15
	An excellent remedy for eye troubles.	
2.	Alum Root	10
	Astringent; tonic.	

3.	Red Oak Bark	10
	Astringent.	
		OUNCES
4.	Distilled Water	2
		GRAINS
5.	Boric Acid	15
	Detergent wash; antiseptic.	
6.	Zinc Sulfate Powder	1
	Astringent.	
7.	Camphor	½
	Soothing to the nerves; antiseptic.	

Boil nos. 1, 2, and 3 in 2 ounces of distilled water slowly down to 1 ounce; strain. Dissolve nos. 5, 6, and 7 in the decoction while still warm, let stand for a few hours, then filter through filter paper.

Directions: Place 2 or 3 drops into eye two or three times a day.

This formula is very soothing and cleansing to watery, inflamed, weak, and tired eyes, and can also be used after removing foreign bodies from the eyes.

NO. 45
Foot Powder

		OUNCES	APPROX. EQUIV.
1.	Club Moss	⅛	¼ Tbsp.
	Dusting powder; promotes healing.		
2.	Sodium Borate (Borax)	1¼	2½ Tbsp.
	Cleansing agent.		
3.	Purified Talc	1¼	2½ Tbsp.
	Protective and soothing powder.		
4.	Zinc Sulfate	⅛	¼ Tbsp.
	Astringent; disinfectant.		

123

		DROPS	
5.	Eugenol (from Oil of Cloves)	10	10 drops
	Antiseptic; counterirritant.		
6.	Formaldehyde	5	5 drops
	Reduces perspiration; disinfectant.		

Mix well and pass through a sieve of small mesh.

Directions: Dust on feet freely and place some of the powder in the socks before putting them on. This should be done morning and night. The mild yet efficient action of No. 45 is very gratifying to those who suffer from perspiring, burning, and sore feet. It not only acts as a soothing agent, but neutralizes bad odors as well.

As cleanliness is one of the main factors in overcoming this trouble, it is advisable to use a foot bath every night before retiring. No. 46 will be found of special benefit in toning and strengthening the tissues of the feet. A little of the foot powder (No. 45) should be sprinkled on the feet after the foot bath.

NO. 46
Herbs for Foot Bath

		OUNCES	APPROX. EQUIV.
1.	Wild Sage	1	2 Tbsp.
	Relieves inflammation.		
2.	Red Oak Bark	3	6 Tbsp.
	Contracts swollen tissues.		
3.	Soap Bark	1	2 Tbsp.
	Makes a lather.		
4.	Snake Plantain	1	2 Tbsp.
	Promotes healing; astringent.		

Mix well, using herbs especially cut for tea.

Directions: Take 3 tablespoonfuls of the mixed herbs and 2 tablespoonfuls of borax (to soften the water) and place in water of sufficient quantity to make a foot bath. Boil slowly for about 5 minutes, then strain and soak the feet in the decoction for about 10 minutes.

NO. 47
Bile Capsules

		GRAINS
1.	Menthol	10
	Relieves nausea and spasms.	
2.	Bile Salts	60
	Stimulates intestinal activity and the flow of bile.	
3.	Aloe	60
	Effects copious stools; increases peristalsis.	

Mix well, using finely powdered material. Divide into 35 equal doses and fill capsules.

Directions: One or two capsules before retiring.

The action of this recipe helps to remove catarrhal slime from stomach and bowels, increases the flow of bile, and stimulates the activity of the bowels and liver. In order to obtain the best results, these capsules should be taken over a period of time.

This recipe is of special benefit in liver and gallbladder complaints, and in constipation due to sluggishness of the liver. Where a catarrhal, congested, or obstructed condition of the gallbladder exists, No. 48 should be taken.

NO. 48
Gallbladder Remedy

	OUNCES
1. Best Lucca Gum Oil	5
Loosens obstructions; causes flow of bile.	
2. Distilled Water	1
Solvent for the salts.	

	GRAINS
3. Sodium Oleate	5
Induces peristalsis; increases the discharge of bile.	
4. Aromatics to flavor	As desired
To improve the taste of this preparation.	

Dissolve no. 3 in no. 2, then add nos. 1 and 4 and shake until a uniform emulsion is obtained.

Directions: Take two capsules of No. 47 half an hour before taking No. 48. The entire contents of No. 48 should be poured into a cup (diluted with water if desired) and taken all in one dose. This preparation should be taken on an evening when the patient does not work the following day, as the contents of the stools for the next 24 hours must be watched. Because of the size of the dose there may be some nausea, but it is perfectly harmless and safe. In such cases a small quantity of lemon or orange juice may be taken. The best way of examining the stools is by using either a bedpan or pail and washing the stools with water. All congealed bile, which is light and waxy, will float on top, and matter of a calcareous nature will sink to the bottom. If the trouble is due to catarrh, catarrhal slime will be found in the stools. No. 48 should be repeated once a week until stools are found to be normal. No. 47, however, should be taken regularly as long as the bowels need regulation.

No. 48 has saved thousands from gallbladder operations. It is harmless and safe. It removes obstructions without pain and should be given a fair trial before resorting to an operation.

NO. 49
Urinary Antiseptic

		DRACHMS	APPROX. EQUIV.
1.	Buchu Leaves An effective urinary antiseptic; relieves inflammation.	4	4 tsp.
2.	Uva Ursi Leaves Very valuable in catarrhal inflammation of the urinary tract.	6	6 tsp.
3.	Sweet Fern A mild but effective diuretic.	3	3 tsp.
4.	Hydrangea Leaves Relieves inflammation of urinary canal and bladder.	3	3 tsp.
5.	Blue Flag A valuable diuretic; cleanses the mucous lining.	2	2 tsp.
6.	Trailing Arbutus A very useful urinary antiseptic and astringent.	6	6 tsp.
7.	Scouring Rush Heals and soothes the inflamed tissues.	6	6 tsp.

Mix well and divide into 20 doses, using herbs either especially cut for tea or in the powdered form.

Directions for Tea: Add one dose to 3 cups boiling water, cover, boil slowly for about 2 to 3 minutes, let it stand for 10 minutes, then strain and take one third morning, noon, and night, either before or after meals. If boiling water is not available, use hot water and allow to stand for half an hour. It may be sweetened with honey, rock candy, sugar, etc., to suit taste.

Directions for Powder: Divide one dose in three parts, taking one

third morning, noon, and night, either before or after meals. It may be taken in water, or mixed with honey, jelly, or jam.

NO. 50
Urinary Antiseptic Capsules

		DRACHMS	APPROX. EQUIV.
1.	Catechu Powder	1¼	1¼ tsp.
	Arrests mucous discharges.		
2.	Cubeb Berries Powder	2	2 tsp.
	Useful in genito-urinary infections.		
3.	Kava Kava Root	2	2 tsp.
	Urinary antiseptic; relieves pain.		
4.	Button Snakeroot	1	1 tsp.
	Relieves inflammation and pain.		
5.	Balsam Copaiba	3¾	3¾ tsp.
	Diminishes unnatural discharges.		
		DROPS	
6.	Oil of Lovage	4	4 drops

Make into a paste. Divide into 60 equal doses and fill capsules. *Directions:* One capsule three times a day after meals, with water.

NO. 51
For Gout

		DRACHMS	APPROX. EQUIV.
1.	Prickly Ash Bark	2	2 tsp.
	Cleanses liver and blood.		

2.	Buckthorn Bark	5	5 tsp.
	Regulates the bowels and cleanses the system.		
3.	Black Cohosh Root	6	6 tsp.
	Relieves acid conditions of the blood.		
4.	Bitter Root	6	6 tsp.
	Reduces rheumatic accumulations.		
5.	Colchicum Seeds	1	1 tsp.
	Has a specific action in gout and rheumatism.		
6.	Bittersweet Twigs	2	2 tsp.
	Relieves inflammation in gout and rheumatism.		
7.	Licorice	4	4 tsp.
	Has a mild laxative effect.		
8.	Buckbean Leaves	4	4 tsp.
	Aids the excretion of acid.		

Mix well and divide into 20 doses, using herbs either especially cut for tea or in the powdered form.

Directions for Tea: Add one dose to 3 cups of boiling water, cover, boil slowly for about 2 to 3 minutes, let it stand for 10 minutes, then strain and take one third morning, noon, and night, either before or after meals. If boiling water is not available, use hot water and allow to stand for half an hour. It may be sweetened with honey, rock candy, sugar, etc., to suit taste.

Directions for Powder: Divide one dose in three parts, taking one third morning, noon, and night, either before or after meals. It may be taken in water or mixed with honey, jelly, or jam.

NO. 52

Herb Vinegar for External Use

		DRACHMS	APPROX. EQUIV.
1.	Belladonna Leaves	6	6 tsp.
	Relieves pain; quiets the nervous system.		
2.	Black Henbane Leaves	6	6 tsp.
	Relieves pain and spasms; quiets nerves.		
3.	Peppermint Leaves	2	2 tsp.
	Quiets spasmodic tendency; stimulates proper function of affected parts.		
4.	Rosemary Leaves	2	2 tsp.
	Quiets the affected nerves.		
5.	Lavender Flowers	2	2 tsp.
	Stimulates proper function; sweet scent.		
6.	Arnica Flowers	2	2 tsp.
	Soothing; counterirritant.		
7.	Cloves	2	2 tsp.
	Stimulates the affected tissues.		
8.	Menthol	½	½ tsp.
	Depresses pain perception.		
9.	Spirit of Camphor	6	6 tsp.
	Stimulates tissues.		
		QUART	
10.	Best Cider Vinegar or Malt Vinegar	1	1 quart

Extract the herbs (nos. 1 through 7) in the vinegar for 4 to 5 days, then strain and add no. 8 dissolved in no. 9.

Directions: Dilute 1 tablespoonful of herb vinegar with a tumbler of cold water and use as cooling compresses frequently until inflammation is relieved.

This is a very useful preparation in all cases where inflammation causes swelling and pain; it acts as a soothing and healing agent.

NO. 53
For Hoarseness

		DRACHMS	APPROX. EQUIV.
1.	Pimpernel Root	6	6 tsp.
	Relieves hoarseness and soreness in throat.		
2.	Marsh Mallow Root	2	2 tsp.
	Acts soothing and healing on mucous membrane.		
3.	Elecampane Root	2	2 tsp.
	Allays coughs and irritations.		
4.	Wild Sage	2	2 tsp.
	Acts as an astringent.		
5.	Licorice	6	6 tsp.
	A helpful expectorant.		
6.	Fennel Seed	2	2 tsp.
	Relieves irritation from coughing.		

Mix well and divide into 20 doses, using herbs especially cut for tea.

Directions: Add one dose to 3 cups boiling water, cover, boil slowly for about 2 or 3 minutes, let it stand for 10 minutes, then strain and take one third morning, noon, and night, either before or after meals. If boiling water is not available, use hot water and allow to stand for half an hour. It may be sweetened with honey, rock candy, sugar, etc., to suit taste.

Pimpernel root is one of the most reliable and harmless remedies that acts as a soothing agent in hoarseness. It is claimed to have a specific action on the vocal cords and can also be used by chewing the root and swallowing the saliva.

NO. 54
For Blood Purifying, No. 1—Mild

(This formula is best suited for those who are not constipated.)

		DRACHMS	APPROX. EQUIV.
1.	Buckthorn Bark	6	6 tsp.
	Cleanses and regulates the system.		
2.	Burdock Root	2	2 tsp.
	Increases secretions.		
3.	Yellow Dock	2	2 tsp.
	Promotes glandular and cellular action.		
4.	Sarsaparilla Root	2	2 tsp.
	Cleanses the blood.		
5.	Pansy Herb	2	2 tsp.
	Beneficial in skin diseases due to impure blood.		
6.	Crimson Clover Blossoms	2	2 tsp.
	Highly praised in ill-conditioned-skin eruptions.		
7.	Licorice Root	3	3 tsp.
	Mild laxative.		
8.	Coriander Seed	1	1 tsp.
	Stimulant; relieves gas.		

Mix well and divide into 20 doses, using herbs either especially cut for tea or in the powdered form.

Directions for Tea: Add one dose to 3 cups boiling water, cover, boil slowly for about 2 to 3 minutes, let it stand for 10 minutes, then strain and take one third morning, noon, and night, either before or after meals. If boiling water is not available, use hot water and allow to stand for half an hour. It may be sweetened with honey, rock candy, sugar, etc., to suit taste.

Directions for Powder: Divide one dose in three parts, taking one

third morning, noon, and night, either before or after meals. It may be taken with water or mixed with honey, jelly, or jam.

NO. 55
For Blood Purifying, No. 2—Strong

(This formula is best suited for those who are inclined to be constipated.)

		DRACHMS	APPROX. EQUIV.
1.	Sassafras Bark	4	4 tsp.
	Refreshes the blood.		
2.	Buckthorn Bark	6	6 tsp.
	Valuable laxative in habitual constipation.		
3.	Crimson Clover Blossoms	2	2 tsp.
	Highly valued in skin eruptions.		
4.	Dandelion Root	5	5 tsp.
	Cleanses the blood by acting on the liver.		
5.	Licorice Root	4	4 tsp.
	Mild laxative.		
6.	Poke Root	2	2 tsp.
	Incites glandular action; regulates and cleanses the system.		
7.	Senna Fruit	6	6 tsp.
	Stimulates the action of the bowels.		
8.	Anise Seed	1	1 tsp.
	Corrects griping and relieves gas.		

Mix well and divide into 20 doses, using herbs either especially cut for tea or in the powdered form.

Directions: Follow the same directions as in No. 54.

These two recipes, Nos. 54 and 55, will be found very beneficial in diseases arising from impure blood, as in pimples, boils, itching skin, and other skin eruptions. They tone and cleanse the system by inciting a healthy action of the glands and blood-building organs, excreting impurities and morbid matter in a natural way.

NO. 56
Scabies Ointment

		DRACHMS	APPROX. EQUIV.
1.	Hellebore Root Powder, American	1	1 tsp.
	Quiets the nervous system.		
2.	Flowers of Sulfur	5	5 tsp.
	Kills parasites.		
3.	Zinc Sulfate	2½	2½ tsp.
	Astringent and disinfectant.		
4.	Gum Storax	2½	2½ tsp.
	Antiseptic against scabies.		
5.	Green Soap	6	6 tsp.
	Softens and stimulates skin.		
6.	Castor Oil	8	8 tsp.
	Softens and soothes tissues.		
7.	Cottonseed Oil	16	16 tsp.
	Gently stimulating to skin.		

Make into a smooth ointment.

Directions: Take a bath as hot as can be comfortably borne before going to bed, and wash all the affected parts with tincture of green soap and water, scrubbing well to open the burrows of the parasites. Then rub in the ointment, taking special care that all affected parts are thoroughly saturated with it. Continue this for three or four nights. Do not change underwear, bed sheets, etc., until the itching has entirely ceased, but afterward be sure to disinfect or boil everything the patient came in contact with. If special care is taken that this ointment is rubbed in thoroughly and the instructions carefully followed, the annoying trouble should disappear within three to four days.

NO. 57
Renal Tea for Kidney Irregularities

		DRACHMS	APPROX. EQUIV.
1.	Button Snakeroot	3	3 tsp.
	Valued in kidney disease.		
2.	Pipsissewa Herb	3	3 tsp.
	Relieves irritation of the entire urinary tract.		
3.	Couch Grass	6	6 tsp.
	Acts soothing and healing on the kidneys.		
4.	Uva Ursi Leaves	8	8 tsp.
	Gives tone to the urinary organs.		
5.	Buchu	5	5 tsp.
	Relieves irritation from kidneys and bladder.		
6.	Juniper Berries	3	3 tsp.
	Regulates the flow of urine.		
7.	Celery Seed	1	1 tsp.
	Acts as a mild diuretic and urinary antiseptic.		
8.	Lovage Root	1	1 tsp.
	Relieves tendency to spasms and cramps.		

Mix well and divide into 20 doses, using herbs either especially cut for tea or in the powdered form.

Directions for Tea: Add one dose to 3 cups boiling water, cover, boil slowly for about 2 to 3 minutes, let it stand for 10 minutes, then

strain and take one third morning, noon, and night, either before or after meals. If boiling water is not available, use hot water and allow to stand for half an hour. It may be sweetened with honey, rock candy, sugar, etc., to suit taste.

Directions for Powder: Divide one dose in three parts, taking one third morning, noon, and night, either before or after meals. It may be taken in water or mixed with honey, jelly, or jam.

This recipe has a very healing and strengthening action upon the kidneys, helping them to function normally. It tends to diminish the quantity of albumin and aids in overcoming the weakening effects of kidney diseases.

NO. 58
Herbs for Douche

		OUNCES	APPROX. EQUIV.
1.	Black Birch Leaves Contracts tissues.	1	2 Tbsp.
2.	Wild Sage Astringent; reduces inflammation.	1	2 Tbsp.
3.	Snake Plantain Soothing and healing; astringent.	1	2 Tbsp.
4.	Canada Fleabane Astringent; tonic to the tissues.	1	2 Tbsp.
5.	Red Oak Bark Astringent.	4	8 Tbsp.
6.	Soap Bark Makes a lather.	2	4 Tbsp.

Mix well and divide into 20 doses, using herbs especially cut for tea.

Directions: Add one dose to a quart of boiling water, boil slowly for 5 minutes, strain when lukewarm, and use as a douche before retiring.

This recipe is a safe and effective preparation for the treatment of vaginal excretions, such as leukorrhea, vaginal catarrh, and other abnormal discharges. It is a mild astringent and deodorant, acts in a soothing and healing manner on the mucous membrane without causing irritation or pain, and can be used for any length of time.

NO. 59
For Measles

		DRACHMS	APPROX. EQUIV.
1.	Saffron, American	4	4 tsp.
	A specific action in measles is claimed for this useful flower.		
2.	Lemon Balm	1	1 tsp.
	Produces sweating and reduces fever.		
3.	Licorice	2	2 tsp.
	Relieves cough and facilitates expectoration.		
4.	Elder Blossoms	2	2 tsp.
	Stimulates the organs of secretion.		
5.	Violet Leaves	1	1 tsp.
	Cleans the blood and aids elimination.		

Mix well and divide into 10 doses, using herbs especially cut for tea.

Directions: Add one dose to 3 cups boiling water, cover, boil slowly for 2 to 3 minutes, let it stand for 10 minutes, then strain and take one third morning, noon, and night, either before or after meals. If boiling water is not available, use hot water and allow to stand for half an hour. It may be sweetened with honey, rock candy, sugar, etc., to suit taste.

NO. 60
Female Regulator Tea No. 1

		DRACHMS	APPROX. EQUIV.
1.	Pennyroyal	8	8 tsp.
	Aids in the menstrual flow.		
2.	Rosemary Leaves	2	2 tsp.
	Relieves cramps, induces menstrual flow.		
3.	Tansy	8	8 tsp.
	Promotes the flow in suppressed menstruation.		
4.	Rue Herb	2	2 tsp.
	Relieves congestion in female organs due to nervousness.		
5.	Blue Cohosh	6	6 tsp.
	Soothes pain in periodic disorders.		
6.	Valerian Root	4	4 tsp.
	Quiets the nerves; relieves spasms.		

Mix well and divide into 20 doses, using herbs especially cut for tea.

Directions: Add one dose to 3 cups boiling water, cover, boil slowly for about 2 to 3 minutes, let it stand for 10 minutes, then strain and take one third morning, noon, and night, either before or after meals. If boiling water is not available, use hot water and allow to stand for half an hour. It may be sweetened with honey, rock candy, sugar, etc., to suit taste.

NO. 61
Female Regulator Tea No. 2

(For painful and spasmodic menstruation.)

		DRACHMS	APPROX. EQUIV.
1.	Blue Cohosh	4	4 tsp.
	Indian remedy to facilitate menstruation.		
2.	Nerve Root	4	4 tsp.
	Stimulates the nervous system.		
3.	Cramp Bark	8	8 tsp.
	Relaxes spasms; relieves cramps.		
4.	Life Root Herb	4	4 tsp.
	Promotes menstrual flow.		
5.	Scullcap	4	4 tsp.
	Quiets the nerves; relieves cramps.		
6.	Figwort	4	4 tsp.
	Relieves pain in difficult menstruation.		

Mix well and divide into 20 doses, using herbs especially cut for tea.

Directions: Same as No. 60.

NO. 62
Female Regulator Tea No. 3

(For profuse menstruation.)

		DRACHMS	APPROX. EQUIV.
1.	Button Snakeroot	6	6 tsp.
	Gives tone and energy to the uterus.		

139

		DRACHMS	APPROX. EQUIV.
2.	Beth Root	6	6 tsp.
	Strengthens the female reproductive organs.		
3.	Alum Root	4	4 tsp.
	Powerful astringent; arrests bleeding.		
4.	Blue Cohosh	6	6 tsp.
	Stimulates normal contraction of the uterus.		
5.	Canada Fleabane	4	4 tsp.
	Arrests hemorrhages; contracts tissues.		
6.	Shepherd's Purse Herb	4	4 tsp.
	Promotes contraction of blood vessels; stops bleeding.		

Mix well and divide into 20 doses, using herbs especially cut for tea.

Directions: Same as No. 60.

Abnormal functions of the female organs during menstruation often lead to other annoying disturbances, such as headaches, depression, excitability, and restlessness. If these symptoms can be traced to other than menstrual irregularities, then the underlying cause should be removed without delay. In such instances, to resort to headache powders, sleeping powders, or nerve sedatives, which are harmful, merely treats the symptoms, but doesn't effect a cure.

NO. 63
Herb Mixture for Moths

		DRACHMS	APPROX. EQUIV.
1.	Patchouly Leaves	8	8 tsp.
	Moth expellant.		
2.	Tansy	2	2 tsp.
	Repels insects.		

3.	Rosemary	2	2 tsp.
	Aids in insect control.		
4.	Lavender Flowers	4	4 tsp.
	Fragrant scent.		

Mix well and use to fill small muslin bags.

Directions: Hang bags in the closet or lay between sheets in the dresser.

This herb mixture has proven more effective than camphor and mothballs in keeping moths away. Its greatest advantage is that it imparts a refreshing, pleasant, and fragrant odor to the linen and clothing.

NO. 64
Oil for Catarrh

		GRAINS
1.	Menthol	8
	Cooling sensation; depresses pain perception.	
2.	Camphor	8
	Promotes blood flow to affected tissues.	
		DROPS
3.	Oil of Cloves	1
	Stimulates affected tissues.	
4.	Oil of Thyme	1
	Stimulates respiratory organs.	
5.	Oil of Eucalyptus	4
	Stimulating expectorant.	
		GRAINS
6.	Ephedrine	25
	Dilates bronchial ducts.	
7.	Alkanet Root Extract	2
	Astringent; coloring agent.	

OUNCES

8. Mineral Oil   8
    Soothes and reduces inflammation of
    upper respiratory tract.

Dissolve nos. 1, 2, and 6 in no. 8 by the aid of heat, then add nos. 3, 4, 5, and 7.

Directions: Spray by means of an oil atomizer into nostrils and throat morning and night; more often if necessary. The exceedingly fine distribution obtained by the spray carries it to all the parts of the nose and throat, an accomplishment not readily attained by any other method of application. If an atomizer is not at hand, it may be administered to the nostrils with an eye dropper.

This is a very effective recipe for quickly clearing the air passages of the nose and throat. As catarrhal conditions are often responsible for affections and congestion of bronchial tubes and hardness of hearing, it can be used also to advantage in these conditions.

NO. 65
Catarrh Balsam

GRAINS

1. Menthol   5
    Depresses pain perception; cooling sensation.

MINIMS

2. Eucalyptol   5
    Stimulating expectorant.

GRAINS

3. Blood Root Fine Powder   2½
    Expectorant.

4. Galanga Fine Powder   5
    Stimulates affected organs.

		DRACHMS
5.	Healing Balsam (No. 89)	4
	Healing and soothing.	
6.	Yellow Petrolatum	4
	Protective dressing.	

Make into a smooth, uniform salve.

Directions: Apply a small quantity to the mucous membrane of the nose, morning and night.

In mild, temporary cases, and especially in such cases where the catarrhal condition is confined only to the mucous membrane of the nose, this recipe will be found to be effective and reliable.

NO. 66
Nerve Restorative Tea No. 1

		DRACHMS	APPROX. EQUIV.
1.	Scullcap	4	4 tsp.
	A valuable nerve stimulant; produces sleep.		
2.	Valerian Root	12	12 tsp.
	Quiets and strengthens the nervous system.		
3.	Nerve Root	6	6 tsp.
	Relieves nervous tension.		
4.	Rosemary Leaves	2	2 tsp.
	Revives nerve action.		
5.	Lemon Balm	3	3 tsp.
	Soothes and refreshes the nerves.		
6.	Celery Seed	3	3 tsp.
	Tonic and nerve stimulant.		

Mix well and divide into 20 doses, using herbs especially cut for tea.

Directions: Add one dose to 3 cups boiling water, cover, boil slowly for about 2 to 3 minutes, let it stand for 10 minutes, then strain and take one third morning, noon, and night, either before or after meals. If boiling water is not available, use hot water and allow to stand for half an hour. It may be sweetened with honey, rock candy, sugar, etc., to suit taste.

Where the nervous condition is due to female complaints, No. 67 should be used.

NO. 67
Nerve Restorative Tea No. 2

		DRACHMS	APPROX. EQUIV.
1.	Motherwort	6	6 tsp.
	Relieves pains and nerve tension due to female complaints.		
2.	Buckbean	4	4 tsp.
	Gives tone to the nervous system.		
3.	Partridge Berry Herb	4	4 tsp.
	Relieves nervous irritation originating with female irregularities.		
4.	Cramp Bark	4	4 tsp.
	Stimulates the nerve centers controlling the female organs.		
5.	Cassia Bark	4	4 tsp.
	Stimulates the circulatory system.		
6.	Valerian	8	8 tsp.
	Quiets and strengthens the nervous system; induces sleep.		

Mix well and divide into 20 doses, using herbs especially cut for tea.

Directions: The same as No. 66.

It is often advisable to have a reliable and harmless nerve medicine ready for use at any time; the following recipe, No. 68, is given to meet that requirement.

NO. 68
Nerve Restorative Capsules

		GRAINS	APPROX. EQUIV.
1.	Gum Asafetida	30	½ tsp.
	A valuable nerve stimulant, especially in nervous dyspepsia.		
2.	Musk Root Extract	15	¼ tsp.
	Invigorates the nervous system.		
3.	Yellow Ladies' Slipper Root Powder	20	⅓ tsp.
	Relieves nerve pain; induces sleep.		
4.	Peony Root, Powdered	30	½ tsp.
	Stimulates the nerves.		
5.	Scullcap	15	¼ tsp.
	A valuable nerve tonic.		
6.	Valerian Powder	40	⅔ tsp.
	Strengthening and soothing on the nerves.		
		DROPS	
7.	Oil of Celery	7	7 drops
	Quiets the nerves.		

Mix well. Divide into 30 equal doses and fill capsules.
Directions: One capsule three times a day after meals.
This recipe will be found to act promptly and effectively. It aids

145

in imparting strength and vitality to the weakened nervous system. It is an invaluable aid in nervousness, sleeplessness, restlessness, excitability, and nervous exhaustion.

NO. 69
Analgesic Balm

		DRACHMS	APPROX. EQUIV.
1.	Henbane Leaves Fluidextract	½	½ tsp.
	Relieves pain; calms the nerves.		
2.	Belladonna	½	½ tsp.
	Relieves pain; depresses nerves.		
3.	Oil of Rosemary	½	½ tsp.
	Soothes affected nerves.		
4.	Oil of Thyme	½	½ tsp.
	Stimulates affected tissues.		
5.	Oil of Lavender	½	½ tsp.
	Aromatic stimulant.		
6.	Oil of Broom Pine	2	2 tsp.
	Counterirritant.		
7.	Oil of Bay Laurel Berries	2½	2½ tsp.
	Aromatic stimulant.		
8.	Oil of Black Mustard	1/10	6 drops
	Increases blood flow to affected parts.		
9.	Gum Camphor	⅓	⅓ tsp.
	Stimulates blood flow.		
10.	Menthol	½	½ tsp.
	Depresses pain perception.		
11.	Healing Balsam, No. 89	8	8 tsp.
	Soothing and healing.		

Make into a smooth ointment.

Directions: Apply to affected parts morning and night, and oftener if necessary.

Sometimes an external pain-relieving remedy is desirable to get quick relief from nerve pains, neuralgia, nervous headache, or congestion in the head. No. 69, applied by rubbing into the affected parts, will be found very effective for that purpose. It invigorates and stimulates the nerves, relieves congestion, and allays pain and strain.

NO. 70
Smelling Salts

		DRACHMS	APPROX. EQUIV.
1.	Ammonium Carbonate Crystals Nasal stimulant.	4	4 tsp.
2.	Stronger Ammonia Water Nasal irritant; stimulant.	¼	¼ tsp.
3.	Spirits of Camphor Stimulant.	½	½ tsp.
		DROPS	
4.	Lavender Oil Aromatic stimulant.	5	5 drops
5.	Ylang-Ylang Perfume.	1	1 drop

Saturate no. 1 with the liquids, and place in a well-stoppered bottle. *Directions:* Inhale gently through the nostrils when needed.

Great benefit and quick results are often obtained from the refreshing and reviving effect of smelling salts. No. 70 is a good recipe and gives almost instant relief in fainting spells, dizziness, simple headache, nervous weakness, and similar conditions. It should always be at hand wherever these conditions prevail.

NO. 71
Herb Health Tea

		OUNCES	APPROX. EQUIV.
1.	Red Clover Blossoms	6	12 Tbsp.
	An effective blood purifier.		
2.	Anise Seed	4	8 Tbsp.
	An aromatic tonic.		
3.	Damiana Leaves	2	4 Tbsp.
	Invigorates the body and nerves.		
4.	Strawberry Leaves	3	6 Tbsp.
	An effective alkalinizer.		
5.	Woodruff Herb	1	2 Tbsp.
	Aids digestion; quiets the nerves.		

Mix well, using herbs especially cut for tea.

Directions: Prepare like ordinary tea, about a teaspoonful to a cup of boiling water. Do not boil; allow to steep for a few minutes. Sugar, honey, cream, or milk may be added to suit taste. When iced, it makes an invigorating and refreshing summer drink.

Nervous people, and all those who suffer from a rundown condition or stomach disorders, should not use coffee or tea. These tend to irritate the nerves and retard the action of the digestive organs. They should use instead a substitute that will not act as an irritant, such as peppermint, chamomile flowers, linden flowers, maté (South America's national beverage), etc. Still better, a mixture of herbs, such as No. 71, will be found to be a palatable and excellent after-meal beverage.

NO. 72
Neuralgia Anodyne

		DRACHMS	APPROX. EQUIV.
1.	Oil of Wintergreen	½	½ tsp.
	Relieves aches and pains.		
2.	Oil of Cajeput	¼	¼ tsp.
	Counterirritant.		
3.	Oil of Cloves	⅛	⅛ tsp.
	Stimulant.		
4.	Oil of Black Mustard	⅓	⅓ tsp.
	Increases blood flow to affected parts.		
5.	Oleoresin of Cayenne Pepper	¼	¼ tsp.
	Stimulant; increases blood flow to affected parts.		
6.	Campho-Menthol	⅓	⅓ tsp.
	Decreases pain perception.		
7.	Broom Pine Oil	5	5 tsp.
	Counterirritant.		
8.	Chloroform	1¼	1¼ tsp.
	Relieves pain.		

Mix all and shake until dissolved.

Directions: Moisten fingertips or cotton with the liniment and rub well into affected parts.

This is a very good recipe to relieve nerve pains of any kind quickly and effectively, but the trouble itself can only be overcome by removing the underlying cause.

NO. 73
For Neuritis

		DRACHMS	APPROX. EQUIV.
1.	Buckthorn Bark	6	6 tsp.
	Cleanses and regulates the system.		
2.	Cassia Bark	2	2 tsp.
	Gives tone to the circulatory system.		
3.	Black Cohosh Root	8	8 tsp.
	Relieves acid conditions of the blood.		
4.	Yellow Dock Root	4	4 tsp.
	Promotes glandular action; cleanses the blood.		
5.	Poke Root	2	2 tsp.
	Very effective as a system regulator and cleanser.		
6.	Senna Fruit	4	4 tsp.
	Removes accumulations from stomach and bowels.		
7.	Licorice	4	4 tsp.
	Mild laxative.		

Mix well and divide into 20 doses, using herbs either especially cut for tea or in the powdered form.

Directions for Tea: Add one dose to 3 cups boiling water, boil slowly for about 2 to 3 minutes, let it stand for 10 minutes, then strain and take one third morning, noon, and night, either before or after meals. If boiling water is not available, use hot water and allow to stand for half an hour. It may be sweetened with honey, rock candy, sugar, etc., to suit taste.

Directions for Powder: Divide one dose in three parts, taking one third morning, noon, and night, either before or after meals. It may be taken in water or mixed with honey, jelly, or jam.

In all rheumatic conditions affecting the nerves, as in neuritis, neuralgia, and sciatica, this recipe can be used with excellent results. It soothes the pain, reduces the acid content of the blood, promotes glandular action, and invigorates the circulatory system.

NO. 74
For Night Sweats

		DRACHMS	APPROX. EQUIV.
1.	Wild Sage Leaves	12	12 tsp.
	Excellent in checking excessive sweating.		
2.	Rosemary Leaves	2	2 tsp.
	Quiets the nerves; normalizes skin action.		
3.	Buckbean	4	4 tsp.
	Reduces fever; invigorates the system.		
4.	Boneset	2	2 tsp.
	Tones up the system; relieves feverish conditions.		

Mix well and divide into 20 doses, using herbs especially cut for tea.

Directions: Add one dose to a cup of boiling water, let steep for about 5 minutes, then strain and take before retiring.

NO. 75
Herbs for Reducing

		DRACHMS	APPROX. EQUIV.
1.	Sea Wrack	5	5 tsp.
	Provides organic iodine; regulates glandular functions.		

2.	Buckthorn Bark	3	3 tsp.
	Cleanses the system of impurities.		
3.	Senna Fruit	5	5 tsp.
	Stimulates the organs of elimination.		
4.	Chickweed	3	3 tsp.
	Reduces unnatural accumulations of fat.		
5.	Licorice	2	2 tsp.
	Mild laxative.		
6.	Cassia Bark	1	1 tsp.
	Improves the action of the circulatory system.		
7.	Poke Root	1	1 tsp.
	Has a direct action on the glandular system; reduces fat.		

Mix well and divide into 20 doses, using herbs either especially cut for tea or in the powdered form.

Directions for Tea: Add one dose to 3 cups boiling water, cover, boil slowly for about 2 to 3 minutes, let it stand for 10 minutes, then strain and take one third morning, noon, and night, either before or after meals. If boiling water is not available, use hot water and allow to stand for half an hour. It may be sweetened with honey, rock candy, sugar, etc., to suit taste.

Directions for Powder: Divide one dose in three parts, taking one third morning, noon, and night, either before or after meals. It may be taken in water or mixed with honey, jelly, or jam.

The good results obtained from the use of this mixture are due to its properties in normalizing glandular action, which is often responsible for the accumulation of fat. It aids better elimination and supplies organic iodine to the system. Its action is along natural lines and is not injurious.

NO. 76
Capsules for Hemorrhoids

		GRAINS
1.	Mandrake Root Extract Regulates liver and bowels and thus relieves pressure in the rectum.	3
2.	Culver's Root Extract Stimulates the flow of bile.	20
3.	Rhubarb Root Increases muscular action of the bowels.	20
4.	Poke Root Regulates and cleans the system.	20
5.	Scullcap Nerve tonic.	3
6.	Cascara Sagrada Bark Extract Cleans the colon; softens the stools.	40

Mix well, using finely powdered material. Divide into 20 equal doses and fill capsules.

Directions: One capsule before retiring. In stubborn cases of constipation, one capsule morning and night may be taken.

NO. 77
Rectal Wash for Hemorrhoids

		OUNCES	APPROX. EQUIV.
1.	Red Oak Bark Astringent.	1¼	2½ Tbsp.
2.	Willow Bark Astringent; tones the affected tissues.	1½	3 Tbsp.

3.	Wild Sage Leaves	¾	1½ Tbsp.
	Astringent; relieves inflammation.		
4.	Comfrey	¾	1½ Tbsp.
	Astringent.		
5.	Canada Fleabane	¾	1½ Tbsp.
	Astringent.		

Mix well and divide into 20 doses, using herbs especially cut for tea.

Directions: Add one dose to a pint of boiling water, boil slowly for about 2 to 3 minutes, let stand until cold, then strain and use as a rectal enema before retiring.

Where congestion or an inflamed condition in the rectum prevails, enemas acting as a cooling agent are very helpful. Their mild astringent properties act as a soothing and healing agent, relieving heat and pain at the same time. They also tend to remove slime and pressure from the rectum.

NO. 78
Hemorrhoid Cones

		GRAINS
1.	Nutgall Powder	40
	Astringent.	
2.	Canada Fleabane Powder	20
	Astringent.	
3.	Henbane Leaves Powder	24
	Relieves pain; soothes nerves.	
4.	Amaranth Powder	36
	Astringent.	
		DROPS
5.	Oil of Cloves	4
	Counterirritant.	

		DRACHMS
6.	Cacao Butter	5
	Protective cream base for suppositories.	

Mix well and make into 12 suppositories.

Directions: Insert one into rectum before retiring. In more severe cases, one in the morning and one at night may be used.

For the local treatment of hemorrhoids, it is advisable to use suppositories or hemorrhoid cones. They are preferable to salves because they can be easily inserted in the rectum and their quantity is constant. Salves, on the other hand, are hard to administer and the quantity inserted is not definite. No. 78 has been found to give good results as a soothing and healing agent, thus tending to relieve the pain, itching, and inflammation. For best results it should be used persistently, as its action tends to shrink the hemorrhoids gradually.

In order to get the best and quickest results in the treatment of hemorrhoids, the three recipes Nos. 76, 77, and 78 should be used together. No. 76 regulates the bowels and softens the stools, thus relieving the pressure on the hemorrhoids. The wash acts as an effective astringent; it is cooling and healing and keeps the rectum clean. No. 78 (hemorrhoid cones) contains antiseptics, astringents, and soothing agents, thus helping to reduce the enlarged appendages.

NO. 79
Tea for Pleurisy

		DRACHMS	APPROX. EQUIV.
1.	Pleurisy Root	4	4 tsp.
	Facilitates expectoration; loosens phlegm.		
2.	Elecampane Root	3	3 tsp.
	Allays cough and irritation.		
3.	Elder Flowers	2	2 tsp.
	Promotes sweating.		

		DRACHMS	APPROX. EQUIV.
4.	Boneset	2	2 tsp.
	Increases skin action; relieves cough.		
5.	Irish Moss	1	1 tsp.
	A good pectoral stimulant.		
6.	Licorice	3	3 tsp.
	Loosens phlegm from bronchial tubes and lungs.		

Mix well and divide into 10 doses, using herbs especially cut for tea.

Directions: Add one dose to 3 cups boiling water, cover, boil slowly for about 2 to 3 minutes, let it stand for 10 minutes, then strain and take one third morning, noon, and night, either before or after meals. If boiling water is not available, use hot water and allow to stand for half an hour. It may be sweetened with honey, rock candy, sugar, etc., to suit taste.

NO. 80
For Poison Oak and Poison Ivy

		DRACHMS	APPROX. EQUIV.
1.	Grindelia	7	7 tsp.
	Beneficial in poison oak, poison ivy, and other skin irritations.		
2.	Wormwood Herb	2	2 tsp.
	Topical anesthetic in local irritations.		
3.	Soap Bark	5	5 tsp.
	Makes a lather.		
4.	Slippery Elm Bark	4	4 tsp.
	Softens and lubricates skin.		
5.	Wild Sage	2	2 tsp.
	Astringent; relieves inflammation.		

Mix well and divide into 10 doses, using herbs especially cut for tea.

Directions: Add one dose to a pint of boiling water, boil slowly for about 10 minutes, let stand until cool, then strain. Apply cold to affected parts on saturated linens. Continue the application until the swelling is down and the itching has ceased, then apply Healing Balsam, No. 89. This treatment should be kept up until normal condition is restored.

Poultices

Poultices are designed to relieve inflammation and swelling, to allay pain, and to soften and mature boils and ulcers. They are applied hot, about an inch thick, and covered with flannel or a hot-water bag to keep them warm as long as possible.

NO. 81
Poultice Powder

		OUNCES	APPROX. EQUIV.
1.	Slippery Elm Bark Powder	4	8 Tbsp.
	Softens and lubricates skin.		
2.	Fenugreek Seed Powder	4	8 Tbsp.
	Reduces inflammation; forms gummy coating.		
3.	Flax Seed Powder	8	16 Tbsp.
	Softens and soothes tissue; forms gummy coating.		

Mix with hot water or hot milk until a stiff, smooth paste is obtained, and apply to affected parts as described above under "Poultices."

NO. 82
Mustard Poultice

---

1. Black Mustard Powder   1 part
   Relieves rheumatic symptoms by drawing
   blood supply to affected part.
2. Poultice Powder (No. 81)   2 to 3 parts,
   Soothes and softens tissue.   according to effect
                                                              desired.

Directions: Make into a stiff paste with lukewarm water and apply to affected parts as described under "Poultices," p. 157. Leave on for *no more than fifteen minutes,* or less if it causes discomfort.

NO. 83
For Rheumatism

		DRACHMS	APPROX. EQUIV.
1.	Bittersweet Twigs	2	2 tsp.
	Relieves inflammation and pain.		
2.	Prickly Ash Bark	2	2 tsp.
	Very beneficial in rheumatic conditions.		
3.	Poke Root	2	2 tsp.
	Very effective as a system regulator.		
4.	Indian Physic Root	2	2 tsp.
	Reduces rheumatic accumulations.		
5.	Black Cohosh Root	5	5 tsp.
	Indian remedy for rheumatism; relieves pain and irritation.		
6.	Culver's Root	2	2 tsp.
	Liver cleanser and blood purifier.		

7.	Uva Ursi	3	3 tsp.
	Eliminates uric acid by action on the kidneys.		
8.	Meadowsweet	2	2 tsp.
	Increases the flow of urine.		

Mix well and divide into 20 doses, using herbs either especially cut for tea or in the powdered form.

Directions for Tea: Add one dose to 3 cups boiling water, cover, boil slowly for about 2 to 3 minutes, let it stand for 10 minutes, then strain and take one third morning, noon, and night, either before or after meals. If boiling water is not available, use hot water and allow to stand for half an hour. It may be sweetened with honey, rock candy, sugar, etc., to suit taste.

Directions for Powder: Divide one dose in three parts, taking one third morning, noon, and night, either before or after meals. It may be taken in water or mixed with honey, jelly, or jam.

No. 83 has a slight action on the bowels. In the event it should not act sufficiently, No. 25 (System Regulator) should be used in conjunction with it. It is of utmost importance that the bowels be well regulated. The herbs used in this recipe have a tendency to reduce the acid in the system and are therefore highly beneficial in all rheumatic conditions, such as rheumatism, lameness, pain and swelling in the joints, and pain and stiffness in the back, hips, and loins.

NO. 84
Liniment for Rheumatism

		DRACHMS	APPROX. EQUIV.
1.	Mezereon Bark	1	1 tsp.
	Irritant, drawing blood to affected part.		

2.	Cayenne Pepper	2½	2½ tsp.
	Increases blood supply to affected part.		
3.	Alkanet Root	½	½ tsp.
	Coloring agent.		
4.	Oil of Black Mustard	½	½ tsp.
	Relieves rheumatic symptoms by drawing blood to affected part.		
5.	Oil of Rosemary	½	½ tsp.
	Increases blood supply to affected part.		
6.	Oil of Cajeput	½	½ tsp.
	Counterirritant.		
7.	Oil of Wintergreen	2	2 tsp.
	Antirheumatic and counterirritant.		
8.	Oil of Sesame	10	10 tsp.
	Softens skin.		
9.	Gum Camphor	3	3 tsp.
	Increases blood supply to affected part.		
		OUNCES	
10.	Broom Pine Oil	6	12 Tbsp.
	Counterirritant.		

Extract nos. 1, 2, and 3 in nos. 8 and 10 for 2 to 3 days, then filter and add the other ingredients.

Directions: Rub well into affected parts morning and night, more often if necessary.

The deposits of uric acid formed in rheumatic diseases settle easiest and quickest where the circulation is the poorest. It is therefore advisable to use an external application with the internal treatment in order to improve the circulation and draw the blood to the parts that are painful and stiff.

Liniment for Rheumatism, No. 84, will be of great help in promoting better circulation. It helps to relieve the pain, stiffness, lameness, weakness, and swelling of muscles and joints that make rheumatism so unpleasant and troublesome.

This liniment can also be used with good results where a lack of circulation has been caused by a blow, by stretching, twisting, sprains, or bruises, and where stiffness in neck, limbs, and muscles is due to cold.

It must not be overlooked that opening the pores of the skin by sweating is very important in rheumatism. No. 21 or No. 22 should therefore also be used in conjunction with No. 83.

NO. 85
For Sleeplessness

		DRACHMS	APPROX. EQUIV.
1.	Jamaica Dogwood	2½	2½ tsp.
	An effective nerve sedative.		
2.	Scullcap Herb	5	5 tsp.
	Quiets and strengthens the nerves.		
3.	Peony Root	2½	2½ tsp.
	Acts soothing and stimulating on the nerves.		
4.	Linden Flowers	3	3 tsp.
	Tonic and nerve stimulant.		
5.	Celery Seed	2	2 tsp.
	Relieves nerve irritation.		

Mix well and divide into 10 doses.

Directions: Add one dose to a cup of boiling water, boil slowly for a minute or two, let stand from 5 to 10 minutes, then strain and drink before retiring.

NO. 86
Restorative Herb Powder

		GRAINS	APPROX. EQUIV.
1.	Scullcap	20	⅓ tsp.
	A valuable nerve tonic.		
2.	Vanilla Beans	40	⅔ tsp.
	Stimulates the generative system.		
		DRACHMS	
3.	Yohimbé Bark	5	5 tsp.
	Tones the reproductive organs.		
4.	Muirapuama Root	5	5 tsp.
	Invigorates the sexual system.		
5.	Damiana Leaves	3	3 tsp.
	Increases sexual functions.		
6.	Unicorn Root	5	5 tsp.
	Gives tone and energy to the generative organs.		
7.	Cassia Bark	1	1 tsp.
	Tones the circulatory system.		

Mix well, using finely powdered material; divide into 20 powders.
Directions: Take one powder morning and one at night in some water.

NO. 87
Dusting Powder

		DRACHMS	APPROX. EQUIV.
1.	Club Moss	3	3 tsp.
	Promotes healing; dusting powder.		

2.	Calamine	6	6 tsp.
	Drying agent.		
3.	Milk of Sulfur	3	3 tsp.
	Softens horny layer of skin.		
4.	Venice Talcum	20	20 tsp.
	Protective and soothing powder.		
		GRAINS	
5.	Menthol	20	⅓ tsp.
	Depresses pain perception; cools.		
		DROPS	
6.	Oil of Cloves	20	20 drops
	Counterirritant.		

Mix well.
Directions: Dust on affected parts morning and night.

NO. 88
Herbs for Soothing Compresses

		OUNCES	APPROX. EQUIV.
1.	Great Celandine Leaves	½	1 Tbsp.
	Useful in skin diseases.		
2.	Henbane Leaves	½	1 Tbsp.
	Relieves pain; soothes nerves.		
3.	Wild Sage Leaves	1	2 Tbsp.
	Relieves inflammation; astringent.		
4.	Low Mallow Leaves	1	2 Tbsp.
	Softens and soothes tissues.		
5.	Canada Fleabane	1	2 Tbsp.
	Astringent; tones affected tissues.		

Mix well and divide into 10 doses, using herbs especially cut for tea.

Directions: Add one dose to a pint of boiling water, boil slowly for 2 to 3 minutes, let stand until lukewarm, then strain and use cold as compresses on affected parts.

The application of cooling compresses is often advisable; they tend to relieve fever and pain when applied to the affected parts. Good results are obtained from No. 88, which acts as a healing and soothing agent.

NO. 89
Healing Balsam

		DRACHMS	APPROX. EQUIV.
1.	Balm of Gilead Buds	1	1 tsp.
	Promotes healing.		
2.	Marigold Flowers	¼	¼ tsp.
	Promotes healing.		
3.	Colophony (Resin)	3	3 tsp.
	Preservative in ointments.		
4.	White Turpentine	2	2 tsp.
	Local irritant, drawing blood to affected parts.		
5.	Prepared Suet	3	3 tsp.
	Base for ointments.		
6.	Yellow Wax	2	2 tsp.
	Base for ointments.		
7.	Sesame Oil	6	6 tsp.
	Promotes softness of skin.		
8.	Camphor	¼	¼ tsp.
	Increases blood supply to affected parts; antiseptic.		
9.	Eugenol (from Oil of Cloves)	¼	¼ tsp.
	Local irritant, drawing blood to affected parts.		

Melt nos. 3, 4, 5, 6, and 7. Add nos. 1 and 2, let simmer slowly for about 5 minutes, then strain. Finally add nos. 8 and 9, stirring until dissolved, and allow to cool.

Directions: Apply to affected parts two to three times a day.

The healing and soothing properties of this ointment make it very valuable in the treatment of sunburns, burns, scalds; cuts, sores; inflamed, itching, or chapped skin; sore nipples; cold sores, fever blisters, etc.

NO. 90
For Gastritis

		DRACHMS	APPROX. EQUIV.
1.	Buckbean Leaves	4	4 tsp.
	Stimulates digestive activity.		
2.	Yarrow Leaves	2	2 tsp.
	Valuable in flatulent colic.		
3.	Cayenne Pepper	2	2 tsp.
	Aids digestion and assimilation of food.		
4.	Yerba Santa Leaves	2	2 tsp.
	Very useful in catarrhal conditions; removes phlegm.		
5.	Cassia Bark	2	2 tsp.
	Useful aromatic digestive.		
6.	Bitter Root (Gentian)	4	4 tsp.
	Invigorates digestion; relieves gas.		
7.	Licorice	4	4 tsp.
	Loosens slime from mucous membrane.		

Mix well and divide into 20 doses, using herbs either cut for tea or in the powdered form.

Directions for Tea: Add one dose to 3 cups boiling water, cover, boil slowly for about 2 to 3 minutes, let it stand for 10 minutes, then

strain and take one third morning, noon, and night, either before or after meals. If boiling water is not available, use hot water and allow to stand for half an hour. It may be sweetened with honey, rock candy, sugar, etc., to suit taste.

Directions for Powder: Divide one dose in three parts, taking one third morning, noon, and night, either before or after meals. It may be taken in water or mixed with honey, jelly, or jam.

Those objecting to the bitter taste of No. 90 may use the following recipe, No. 91, in capsule form. The ingredients are in a concentrated form, possess powerful digestive properties, and are very effective and prompt in action.

NO. 91
Capsules for Gastritis

		GRAINS	APPROX. EQUIV.
1.	Scullcap Powder	30	½ tsp.
	Quiets nervous activity.		
2.	Papaya Fruit Extract	60	1 tsp.
	A digestive of extraordinary power.		
3.	Malt Diastase Powder	60	1 tsp.
	Increases the digestibility of starches.		
4.	Cayenne Pepper	75	1¼ tsp.
	Aids the assimilation of food.		
5.	Goldenseal Root	75	1¼ tsp.
	Useful in catarrhal affections of the stomach.		

Mix well. Divide into 60 equal doses and fill capsules.

Directions: One capsule three times a day after meals, with some water.

No. 90 and No. 91 will be found very beneficial in catarrhal conditions of the stomach. They are useful and effective in sour and gas conditions of the stomach, and tend to relieve the feeling of fullness and distress after eating. They aid the digestion and assimilation of the food and help in cleaning the mucous membranes of slime and of food that has been retained too long.

NO. 92
For Nervous Dyspepsia

		DRACHMS	APPROX. EQUIV.
1.	Valerian Root	10	10 tsp.
	Quiets and strengthens the nerves controlling the stomach.		
2.	Rue Herb	2	2 tsp.
	Relieves nervous irritation and pain.		
3.	Water Mint Herb	2	2 tsp.
	Aids digestion; relieves gas.		
4.	Cayenne Pepper	2	2 tsp.
	Aids assimilation of food.		
5.	Scullcap Herb	4	4 tsp.
	Relieves nervous irritability.		
6.	St. John'swort Herb	3	3 tsp.
	Stimulates the action of stomach and liver.		
7.	Cassia Bark	2	2 tsp.
	Tones up the circulatory system.		
8.	Licorice	5	5 tsp.
	Loosens mucus from stomach and bowels.		

Mix well and divide into 20 doses, using herbs either especially cut for tea or in the powdered form.

Directions for Tea: Add one dose to 3 cups boiling water, cover, boil slowly for about 2 to 3 minutes, let it stand for 10 minutes, then

strain and take one third morning, noon, and night, either before or after meals. If boiling water is not available, use hot water and allow to stand for half an hour. It may be sweetened with honey, rock candy, sugar, etc., to suit taste.

Directions for Powder: Divide one dose in three parts, taking one third morning, noon, and night, either before or after meals. It may be taken in water or mixed with honey, jelly, or jam.

It is often desirable to have a medicine for dyspepsia ready for immediate use. In such cases, the following recipe, No. 93, in capsule form, will meet this requirement. It is quick and dependable in action.

NO. 93

Capsules for Nervous Dyspepsia

		GRAINS	APPROX. EQUIV.
1.	Valerian Extract	20	⅓ tsp.
	Quiets and strengthens the gastric nerves.		
2.	Asafetida	30	½ tsp.
	Relieves nervous irritability.		
3.	Musk Root Extract	60	1 tsp.
	Has a soothing and healing action on the stomach; relieves gas.		
4.	Nutmeg	30	½ tsp.
	Soothes the nerves controlling stomach activity.		
5.	Scullcap Powder	30	½ tsp.
	Quiets nerve action.		

Mix well, using finely powdered material. Divide into 60 equal doses and fill capsules.

Directions: One capsule three times a day after meals, with some water.

NO. 94
For Ulcers of the Stomach and Duodenum
No. 1

		DRACHMS	APPROX. EQUIV.
1.	Golden Seal Root	4	4 tsp.
	Healing to mucous surfaces and tissues.		
2.	Blood Root	1	1 tsp.
	Creates new and healthy energy.		
3.	Amaranth Leaves	2	2 tsp.
	Useful in ulceration of stomach, mouth, and throat.		
4.	Black Birch Leaves	4	4 tsp.
	Tones stomach and bowels.		
5.	Pansy Leaves	2	2 tsp.
	Disperses ulcers and tumors.		
6.	Cinchona Bark	2	2 tsp.
	An effective digestive tonic with strong antiseptic properties.		
7.	Great Celandine Herb	5	5 tsp.
	Has a healing effect on ulcers and growths.		

Mix well and divide into 20 doses, using herbs either especially cut for tea or in the powdered form.

Directions for Tea: Add one dose to 3 cups boiling water, cover, boil slowly for about 2 to 3 minutes, let it stand for 10 minutes, then strain and take one third morning, noon, and night, either before or after meals. If boiling water is not available, use hot water and allow to stand for half an hour. It may be sweetened with honey, rock candy, sugar, etc., to suit taste.

Directions for Powder: Divide one dose in three parts, taking one third morning, noon, and night, either before or after meals. It may be taken in water or mixed with honey, jelly, or jam.

In case of bleeding from the stomach, the following recipe is preferable.

NO. 95
For Ulcers of the Stomach and Duodenum
No. 2

		DRACHMS	APPROX. EQUIV.
1.	Alum Root	2	2 tsp.
	Powerful astringent; arrests excessive mucous discharges.		
2.	Golden Seal Root	4	4 tsp.
	Healing and soothing to mucous lining.		
3.	Canada Fleabane Herb	2	2 tsp.
	Contracts loose tissues; arrests bleeding.		
4.	Shepherd's Purse Herb	3	3 tsp.
	Contracts blood vessels; stops bleeding.		
5.	Red Oak Bark	4	4 tsp.
	A helpful antiseptic for stomach and bowels.		
6.	Buckbean	2	2 tsp.
	Stimulates the digestive organs.		
7.	Goldthread	2	2 tsp.
	Gives tone to the mucous lining; reduces the tendency to bleed.		
8.	Violet Leaves	3	3 tsp.
	Has a healing effect on ulcers.		

Mix well and divide into 20 doses, using herbs either especially cut for tea or in the powdered form.

Directions: Same as No. 94.

NO. 96
For Stone or Gravel in Kidneys or Bladder

		DRACHMS	APPROX. EQUIV.
1.	Pichi Tops	6	6 tsp.
	A reliable solvent for calcareous deposits.		
2.	Trailing Arbutus	4	4 tsp.
	Very beneficial and effective in gravel.		
3.	Hydrangea	10	10 tsp.
	Highly recommended for the removal of stones and gravel.		
4.	Golden Rod, European	4	4 tsp.
	Useful in urinary obstructions, especially when they cause bleeding.		
5.	Uva Ursi	4	4 tsp.
	Gives tone to the urinary organs.		
6.	Scouring Rush	2	2 tsp.
	Relieves inflammation of the mucous membrane.		

Mix well and divide into 20 doses, using herbs either especially cut for tea or in the powdered form.

Directions for Tea: Add one dose to 3 cups boiling water, cover, boil slowly for about 2 to 3 minutes, let it stand for 10 minutes, then strain and take one third morning, noon, and night, either before or after meals. If boiling water is not available, use hot water and allow to stand for half an hour. It may be sweetened with honey, rock candy, sugar, etc., to suit taste.

Directions for Powder: Divide one dose in three parts, taking one

third morning, noon, and night, either before or after meals. It may be taken in water or mixed with honey, jelly, or jam.

The herbs in this recipe are known for their power to dissolve and remove calcareous deposits from the urinary tract gradually, and to relieve inflammation. They are therefore highly recommended in stones or gravel in kidneys or bladder.

NO. 97
For Tapeworm

		GRAINS
1.	Male Fern Root Extract	60
	Considered a specific for the removal of tapeworm.	
2.	Mandrake Root Extract	1½
	A valuable worm expeller.	
3.	Jalap Root	4
	Acts on bowels, producing watery stools.	
		DROPS
4.	Broom Pine Oil	12
	Useful in the expulsion of worms.	

Mix well. Divide into 6 equal doses and fill gelatine capsules.

Directions: Take one capsule every 10 minutes until all are taken. Examine the stools closely and do not forget that the thinnest part of the worm bears the head. Doctors generally let the patient fast for a day or two before taking tapeworm remedies, but this is unnecessary, because the worm, being a parasite, cannot be starved. This only makes the patient feel weak and nauseated; when he finally takes the medicine on a starved stomach, he may vomit it up. A far better way is to advise the patient to eat, for a day or so, foods the tapeworm dislikes, such as onions, garlic, pickles, and salted fish. This weakens the worm and tends to loosen its grip, so that when the medicine is taken, it acts upon the tapeworm and causes it to be expelled more easily.

NO. 98
For Gargle and Mouthwash

		DRACHMS	APPROX. EQUIV.
1.	Wild Sage Leaves Expectorant; relieves inflammation.	10	10 tsp.
2.	Marsh Rosemary Astringent.	10	10 tsp.
3.	Goldthread An astringent especially valued for canker sores.	2	2 tsp.
4.	Rhatany Root Astringent and tonic to the tissues.	2	2 tsp.
5.	Cranesbill Root (Wild Geranium) Astringent and tonic to the tissues.	6	6 tsp.
6.	Red Oak Bark Astringent; mild antiseptic.	6	6 tsp.
7.	Comfrey Root An aromatic stimulant.	2	2 tsp.
8.	Cloves Stimulant.	2	2 tsp.

Mix well and divide into 10 doses, using herbs especially cut for tea.

Directions: Add one dose to a pint of boiling water, boil slowly for 5 minutes, let stand for about 10 minutes, then strain and add 1 tablespoon of table salt to the decoction. Use as a gargle and mouthwash every 2 to 3 hours, until the inflammation and swelling have subsided. If the decoction is found too astringent, it may be diluted with water.

For canker sores may be used externally.

The astringent and antiseptic properties of this recipe make it a very valuable remedy, not only in sore throat, but also in spongy, bleeding gums, canker sores, and bad breath. It is very healing, soothing, and strengthening to the diseased tissues.

NO. 99
For Warts

	GRAINS	APPROX. EQUIV.
1. Trichloracetic Acid Caustic; destroys growths.	15	¼ tsp.
	DROPS	
2. Eugenol (from Oil of Cloves) Local irritant.	5	5 drops
	DRACHMS	
3. Corn Paint (No. 29) For removal of hardened skin lesions.	1¾	1¾ tsp.

Mix well.

Directions: Apply with a glass rod to the warts morning and night; repeat until the destruction of the growth is completed.

NO. 100
Whooping Cough Syrup

	DRACHMS	APPROX. EQUIV.
1. Thyme Leaves Fluidextract Allays irritation; quiets the nerves.	1	1 tsp.
2. Ipecac Root Fluidextract Reliable expectorant.	½	½ tsp.
3. Lobelia Fluidextract Relieves spasms; loosens phlegm.	1½	1½ tsp.

4.	Chestnut Leaves Fluidextract Exerts a specific influence in whooping cough.	1	1 tsp.
		DROPS	
5.	Oil of Wild Thyme Relieves irritation of cough and spasms.	8	8 drops
		DRACHMS	
6.	German Anise Drops Facilitates expectoration; allays cough.	2	2 tsp.
		OUNCES	
7.	Syrup or honey enough to make	8	1 cup

Mix nos. 1 through 6. Add enough no. 7 to equal 8 ounces (1 cup). *Directions:* One teaspoonful every three hours.

As the inhalation of the vapors from soothing balsams is very beneficial, the following recipe is given and may be used with good results in conjunction with this syrup, No. 100.

NO. 101
Inhalation for Whooping Cough

		DRACHMS	APPROX. EQUIV.
1.	Oil of Eucalyptus Stimulating expectorant; germicide; re- lieves fever.	1¼	1¼ tsp.
2.	Oil of Cloves Aromatic stimulant; germicide.	½	½ tsp.
3.	Oil of Pine Needles Expectorant.	1¼	1¼ tsp.
4.	Oil of Broom Pine Counterirritant.	20	20 tsp.

| 5. | Camphor | 1¼ | 1¼ tsp. |

Expectorant; antiseptic.

Mix and shake well until the camphor is dissolved.

Directions: Add 1 teaspoonful of the inhalant to slowly boiling water; allow to evaporate in the patient's room. The vapors purify the air, disinfect the room, ease the attack, and diminish the danger of contagion.

NO. 102
Worm Expeller

		DRACHMS
1.	Pink Root Powder	2
	An excellent destroyer of worms.	
2.	Levant Wormseed Powder	2
	Expels intestinal worms.	
		GRAINS
3.	Santonin	6
	Reputed for its reliable action in expelling worms.	
4.	Mandrake Root Extract	1½
	Acts as a laxative.	

Mix well and divide into 12 powders.

Directions: One powder 3 or 4 times a day, mixed with honey, molasses, or jelly, until all powders are taken.

This treatment should be repeated within a week or so in order to destroy any young worms that may have hatched from eggs left in the intestines before they mature. To relieve the itching in the rectum, injections with warm water in which garlic or onions have been crushed are very beneficial. The outside of the rectum should always be kept clean by washing with soap and water.

NO. 103
Antiseptic Salve

		DRACHMS	APPROX. EQUIV.
1.	Colophony (Resin)	3	3 tsp.
	Preservative in ointments.		
2.	White Turpentine	2	2 tsp.
	Local irritant; antiseptic.		
3.	Yellow Wax	3	3 tsp.
	Ointment base.		
4.	Prepared Suet	8	8 tsp.
	Ointment base.		
5.	Castor Oil	4	4 tsp.
	Softens and soothes the tissue.		
6.	Lanolin	4	4 tsp.
	Ointment base.		
7.	Camphor	½	½ tsp.
	Antiseptic; increases blood supply to affected parts.		
8.	Oil of Cloves	½	½ tsp.
	Germicide.		

Melt all ingredients from no. 1 through no. 6 on a slow fire, then take from the fire. When half cooled, add nos. 7 and 8 and stir until dissolved.

Directions: Apply to affected parts morning and night.

This ointment is especially valuable in the treatment of slow-healing sores, abscesses, ulcers, boils, and carbuncles. It has great healing properties and helps to rebuild the diseased tissues.

4

Key to Medicinal Properties

Alterative: A medicine that alters the process of nutrition and excretion, restoring normal body functions.

Anodyne: Relieving pain.

Anthelmintic: A remedy expelling intestinal worms.

Anti-bilious: Opposing biliousness, acting on the bile.

Anti-epileptic: Opposed to epilepsy, relieves fits.

Anti-fat: An agent that aids in removing excess fat.

Antilithic: Preventing the formation of gravel or stones.

Anti-periodic: Preventing the recurrence of periodic disturbances and irregularities.

Key to Medicinal Properties

Anti-phlogistic: An agent reducing inflammation.

Anti-rheumatic: Correcting and relieving rheumatism.

Antiscorbutic: Preventing or relieving scurvy.

Antiseptic: Preventing or counteracting decay, or the formation of pus.

Antispasmodic: Counteracting or preventing spasms.

Anti-syphilitic: A remedy for the relief of venereal disease.

Aperient: Mild laxative without purging.

Aphrodisiac: Stimulating the sexual passion.

Aromatic: A spicy stimulant.

Astringent: Producing contraction of organic tissue, or the arrest of a discharge.

Carminative: A medicine expelling gases from stomach and bowels.

Cathartic: Producing evacuation from the bowels.

Cholagogue: Promoting and increasing the flow of bile.

Cordial: An aromatic stimulant.

Counterirritant: Causing irritation in one part to relieve pain in another part.

Demulcent: A mucilaginous substance that acts to sooth and relieve inflammation.

Key to Medicinal Properties

Deobstruent: A medicine that removes obstructions.

Depurative: Removing impurities, cleansing the blood.

Detergent: Cleansing to wounds.

Diaphoretic: Producing perspiration.

Discutient: Dispersing tumors and ulcers.

Diuretic: Increasing the secretion and flow of urine.

Drastic: A powerful purgative medicine.

Emetic: Causing vomiting.

Emmenagogue: Promoting and stimulating menstruation.

Emollient: Agent that softens tissue and acts to sooth.

Esculent: Edible as food.

Expectorant: Promoting expelling of mucous secretions from the air passages.

Febrifuge: An agent that lessens fever.

Female Complaint: Disease peculiar to women; therefore, used to describe medicines that cure such diseases.

Female Regulator: An agent that regulates the menstrual flow.

Galactagogue: Increasing the flow of milk.

Hepatic: Promoting the action of the liver and the flow of bile.

Key to Medicinal Properties

Herpetic: An agent useful in diseases of the skin.

Hydragogue: Purgative, causing watery evacuations.

Hypnotic: An agent producing sleep.

Laxative: Producing gentle action of the bowels.

Lithotropic: An agent dissolving stones in the urinary organs.

Mucilaginous: Like mucilage; gummy, viscid.

Narcotic: A hypnotic, inducing stupor.

Nephritic: An agent useful in kidney complaints.

Nervine: An agent calming nervous excitement.

Ophthalmicum: A remedy for diseases of the eye.

Pectoral: A remedy for diseases of chest and lungs.

Poisonous: Producing death, if taken in improper doses.

Pungent: Penetrating or sharp to the taste.

Purgative: A medicine producing watery evacuations.

Saponaceous: Having the nature of soap.

Sedative: An agent allaying irritability.

Sialagogue: Producing a flow of saliva.

Soporific: Producing deep sleep.

Key to Medicinal Properties

Stimulant: An agent increasing functional activity.

Stomachic: Strengthening and giving tone to the stomach.

Stypticum: Arresting hemorrhage or bleeding by causing contraction of the blood vessels.

Sudorific: An agent causing sweating.

Tonic: Producing an increase in the tone of the system.

Vermifuge: An agent expelling intestinal worms.

Vulnerary: An agent favoring the healing of wounds and cuts.

5

Materia Medica Index

Alternatives: Medicines that alter the process of nutrition and excretion, restoring normal body functions.

Barberry Root	Crimson Clover	Sarsaparilla Root
Bittersweet Herb	Fringe Tree Bark	Sassafras Bark
Black Alder Bark	Golden Seal Root	Spikenard Root
Black Cohosh Root	Oregon Grape Root	Wahoo Bark
Buckbean Leaves	Poke Root	Yarrow Herb
Burdock Root	Prickly Ash Bark	Yellow Dock Root
Cinchona Bark	Queen's Root	

Anthelmintics or **Vermifuges:** Medicines expelling intestinal
worms.

Jerusalem Oak	Male Fern Root	Tansy Herb
Flowers	Mandrake Root	Wormseed,
Kamala	Pink Root	American
Koysso Flowers	Pomegranate Bark	
Levant Wormseed	Pumpkin Seeds	

Materia Medica Index

Antilithics: Medicines preventing the formation of gravel and stones.

Buchu Leaves	Pareira Brava Root	Herb
Golden Rod Herb	Pichi Tops	Uva Ursi Leaves
Hydrangea Root	Trailing Arbutus	Violet Leaves

Anti-periodics: Medicines preventing the recurrence of periodic disturbances and irregularities.

Beth Root	Life Root Herb	Rue Herb
Black Willow Bark	Motherwort Herb	Scullcap Herb
Blue Cohosh Root	Partridge Berry	Tansy Herb
Button Snakeroot	Herb	Vervain Herb
Cassia Bark	Pennyroyal Herb	White Poplar Bark
Cramp Bark	Roman Chamomile	
Figwort Herb	Rosemary Leaves	

Anti-rheumatics: Medicines correcting and relieving rheumatism.

Bitter Root	Culver's Root	Poke Root
Bittersweet Twigs	Guaiac Gum	Prickly Ash Bark
Black Alder Bark	Guaiac Wood	Twin Leaf Root
Black Cohosh Root	Kava Kava Root	Virginia Snakeroot
Black Willow Bark	Oregon Grape Root	Yellow Dock Root
Colchicum Seed	Pipsissewa Herb	

Antiseptics: Agents preventing or counteracting decay, or the formation of pus.

Alum Root	Cranesbill Root	Tormentil Root
Amaranth Leaves	Marsh Rosemary	Water Avens Root
Black Alder Bark	Root	Wild Sage Leaves
Black Willow Bark	Oak Bark (Red &	Witch Hazel Herb
Blood Root	White)	
Canada Fleabane	Rhatany Root	

Antispasmodics: Counteracting or preventing spasms.

Beth Root	Black Haw Bark	Chamomile Flowers
Black Cohosh Root	Cassia Bark	Cramp Bark

Antispasmodics: (continued)

Ephedra Herb
Horse Nettle Berries
Indian Turnip Root
Life Root
Linden Flowers
Lobelia Herb
Mistletoe Herb
Motherwort Herb

Mugwort Herb
Mullein Leaves
Nerve Root
Parnassia Herb
Pennyroyal Herb
Peony Root
Pomegranate Bark
Rosemary Leaves

Rue Herb
Scullcap Herb
Valerian Root
Water Mint Herb
White Poplar Bark
Wild Yam Root
Yellow Ladies'
    Slipper Root

Astringents: Agents producing contraction of organic tissues, or the arrest of a discharge.

Alum Root
Amaranth Leaves
Blackberry Root
Black Willow Bark
Canada Fleabane
    Herb
Catechu Gum
Cranesbill Root
Galanga Root
Ginger Root
Goldthread Root

Hydrangea Root
Kino Gum
Lady's Mantle
    Herb
Marsh Rosemary
    Root
Nutgalls
Oak Bark (Red &
    White)
Pomegranate Bark
Rhatany Root

Shepherd's Purse
    Herb
Silver Weed Herb
Tag Alder Bark
Tormentil Root
Water Avens Root
Wild Sage Leaves
Wintergreen Herb
Witch Hazel Herb

Carminatives: Expelling gas from stomach and bowels.

Angelica Root
Angelica Seed
Anise Seed
Canada Snakeroot
Caraway Seed
Cardamom Seed
Catnip Herb

Chamomile
    Flowers, German
Coriander Seed
Cumin Seed
Fennel Seed
Lemon Balm Herb
Lovage Root

Parsley Root
Peppermint Herb
Sweet Flag Root
Thyme Herb
Water Mint Herb
Yerba Buena Herb

Cathartics: Medicines producing evacuations from the bowels.

Balmony Herb
Barberry Bark

Buckthorn Bark
Butternut Bark

Cascara Sagrada
    Bark

Cathartics: (continued)

Culver's Root	Pansy Herb	Senna Leaves
Mandrake Root	Rhubarb Root	Violet Herb

Cholagogues: Medicines promoting and increasing the flow of bile.

Aloe Gum	Great Celandine	Jalap Root
Colycynth Apple	Herb	Mandrake Root
Culver's Root	Hedge Hyssop	Wahoo Bark
Gamboge Gum	Herb	

Coloring Agents: Drugs used in coloring and dyeing.

Alkanet Root (red)	Madder Root (red)	Tartarean Moss
Blood Root (red)	Red Saunders	(purple)
Henna Leaves	Wood (red)	Turmeric Root
(red-brown)	Saffron Flowers	(yellow)
Hollyhock Flowers	(red), American	Walnut Hulls
(wine-red)	Sage Leaves	(brown)
Indigo Leaves	(brown)	
(blue)	Spanish Saffron	
Logwood Chips	(yellow)	
(blue)		

Demulcents: Mucilaginous substances that soothe and relieve inflammation.

Coltsfoot Leaves	Low Mallow Leaves	Plantain Leaves
Comfrey Root	Mallow Leaves	Psyllium Seeds
Fenugreek Seeds	Marsh Mallow	Slippery Elm Bark
Flax Seeds	Root	
Licorice Root	Mullein Leaves	

Depuratives: Removing impurities, cleaning the blood.

Bittersweet Herb	Dulse Leaves	Marsh Rosemary
Buckthorn Bark	Elder Flowers	Root
Burdock Root	Figwort Herb	Meadow Sweet
Culver's Root	Kava Kava Root	Herb
Dandelion Root	Linden Flowers	Oregon Grape Root

Materia Medica Index

Depuratives: (continued)

Pansy Herb
Queen's Root
Red Clover Flowers

Sarsaparilla Root
Sassafras Bark
Senna Fruit

Violet Leaves
Yellow Dock Root

Diaphoretics: Medicines producing perspiration.

Black Birch Leaves
Boneset Herb
Chamomile Flowers
Elder Flowers
Horehound Herb
Jaborandi Leaves

Lemon Balm
   Flowers
Linden Flowers
Pennyroyal Herb
Peppermint Leaves
Pleurisy Root

Vervain Herb
Virginia Snakeroot
Water Mint Herb
Yarrow Herb

Diuretics: Medicines increasing the secretion and flow of urine.

Amaranth Leaves
Black Birch Leaves
Black Indian Hemp
   Root
Broom Tops
Buchu Leaves
Button Snakeroot
Cleavers Herb
Corn Silk
Couch Grass Root
Cubeb Berries
Foxglove Leaves

Golden Rod Herb
Great Celandine
   Herb
Juniper Berries
Kava Kava Root
Lovage Root
Meadow Sweet
   Herb
Parsley Root
Partridge Berry
   Herb
Pichi Leaves

Pipsissewa Herb
Queen of the
   Meadow Root
Scouring Rush
   Herb
Squill Root
Trailing Arbutus
   Herb
Uva Ursi Leaves
Whortleberry
   Leaves

Emetics: Medicines that cause vomiting.

Ipecac Root

Lobelia Herb

Mustard Seed

Emmenagogues: Medicines promoting and stimulating menstruation.

Aloe Gum
Blood Root
Blue Cohosh Root
Cotton Root

Culver's Root
Life Root
Mistletoe Herb
Pennyroyal Herb

Rue Herb
Savin Leaves
Tansy Herb

187

Expectorants: Promoting mucous secretion from the air passages.

Anise Seed	Iceland Moss	Mullein Leaves
Chestnut Leaves	Leaves	Pansy Herb
Coltsfoot Leaves	Ipecac Root	Pleurisy Root
Comfrey Root	Irish Moss	Senega Snakeroot
Elder Flowers	Licorice Root	Soap Bark
Elecampane Root	Lobelia Herb	Squill Root
Fennel Seed	Lungwort Herb	Wild Cherry Bark
Flax Seed	Marsh Mallow	Wild Sage Leaves
Grindelia Herb	Leaves	Wild Thyme Herb
Horehound Herb	Marsh Mallow Root	Yerba Santa Leaves

Febrifuges: Agents that reduce fever.

Aconite Root	Centaury Herb	Virginia Snakeroot
Blood Root	Cinchona Bark	Water Avens Root
Boneset Herb	Dogwood Bark	Yerba Buena Herb
Buckthorn Bark	Quassia Bark	

Hepatics: Promoting action of the liver.

Aloe Gum	Liverwort Herb	Wahoo Bark
Barberry Bark	Mandrake Root	Wild Yam Root
Culver's Root	Poke Root	
Dandelion Root	Rhubarb Root	

Laxatives: Producing gentle action of the bowels.

Balmony Leaves	Dandelion Root	Rhubarb Root
Buckthorn Bark	Mandrake Root	Senna Fruit
Cascara Sagrada	Oregon Grape Root	Senna Leaves
Bark	Pansy Herb	Sloe Tree Flowers
Culver's Root	Poke Root	Wahoo Bark

Nephritics: Agents useful in kidney complaints.

Black Birch Leaves	Button Snakeroot	Juniper Berries
Broom Tops	Couch Grass	Partridge Berry
Buchu Leaves	Root	Herb

Nephritics: (continued)

| Queen of the Meadow Root | Trailing Arbutus Herb | Uva Ursi Leaves Whortleberry Leaves |

Nervines: Medicines that act to calm and sooth the nervous system.

Celery Seed	Musk Root	Scullcap Herb
Cramp Bark	Nerve Root	Valerian Root
Dittany Herb	Peony Root	Yellow Ladies'
Hops	Rosemary Leaves	Slipper Root
Lemon Balm Herb	Rue Herb	

Purgatives: Medicines producing watery evacuations.

Aloe Gum	Cascara Sagrada Bark	Mandrake Root
Black Indian Hemp Root	Colocynth Apple	Rhubarb Root
Buckthorn Bark	Gamboge Gum	Scammony Gum
	Jalap Root	Senna Leaves

Sedatives: Agents allaying irritability.

Aconite Root	Jamaica Dogwood Bark	Water Avens Root
Blood Root	Muirapuama Root	Wild Cherry Bark
Bugleweed Herb	Red Root Bark	Wild Lettuce Leaves
Colchicum Seed	Stramonium Leaves	Yohimbé Bark
Crawley Root	Sweet Fern Leaves	
Foxglove Leaves		
Ice Plant Root		

Stimulants: Medicines increasing functional activity.

Blood Root	Ginger Root	Rosemary Leaves
Cassia Bark	Ginseng Root	Sarsaparilla Root
Damiana Leaves	Linden Flowers	Sassafras Bark
Dandelion Root	Muirapuama Root	Strawberry Leaves
Dwarf Nettle Herb	Prickly Ash Bark	Unicorn Root
Gentian Root	Queen's Root	Valerian Root

Stimulants: (continued)

Wafer Ash Bark   Yellow Dock Root   Yohimbé Bark
Wild Cherry Bark

Vulneraries: Agents favoring the healing of wounds and cuts.

Alum Root   Marsh Rosemary   Poke Root
Arnica Flowers   Root   Rosemary Leaves
Balm of Gilead   Mullein Leaves   Tormentil Root
   Buds   Oak Bark (Red &   Wild Sage Leaves
Cranesbill Root   White)   Witch Hazel
Figwort Herb   Plantain Leaves   Leaves

6

Materia Medica:
The Principal Herbs of Medicinal Value

In the following Materia Medica, we have retained the essence of the original entries as they were written by Otto Mausert. In addition, recent findings from modern science have been added, when available, to provide a more balanced perspective on the herbs.

For dosages of the herbs in this section, we have retained Mausert's original precise measurements. For equivalent measures, see the table of weights and measures in the recipes section, p. 81.

Certain herbs listed in this section have been found to have possible deleterious effects. We therefore recommend caution in the use of any recipes containing these herbs. For minor complaints, there should be a high degree of safety. By no means, however, should any of these herbs, or recipes containing them, be used for any prolonged length of time. The possibly harmful herbs are:

Belladonna
Coltsfoot
Comfrey
Henbane
Mandrake
Pokeberry
Rue
Saint John'swort
Sweet Flag

AGRIMONY
Agrimonia eupatoria; part used: the herb
(German: *Odermennig*   French: *Aigremoine*)
A very valuable herb. It has a tendency to invigorate the functions of stomach, liver, and bowels, eliminating foul matter from the system. It is also highly recommended in the treatment of stones or gravel in kidneys or bladder. As a gargle, the decoction is very effective in soreness and inflammation of mouth and throat.

Recent Findings: Studies in Hong Kong using extracts of the whole plant demonstrated antiviral activity in mice.

Dose: 30–60 grains.

ALOE
Aloe vera and var. spp.;* part used: juice of leaves
(German: *Aloe*   French: *Aloès*   Spanish: *Acibar*)
Aloe is the dried juice of *aloe* leaves. It is a good laxative, promoting and assisting the action of the large intestines. As it also has a tendency to increase the menstrual flow, it should not be used by those who normally have an excessive flow, nor should it be used during the menstrual period or in cases of pregnancy. Sufferers from piles also should avoid it. Its action is milder combined with other medicines and it is preferably used that way.

Recent Findings: The juice of *aloe* leaves, either fresh or in oint-

*var. spp. = various species; several species of this genus are medicinally active.

192

ment form, has emollient properties, and has been used to treat sunburn as well as radiation burns from x rays.

Dose: 3–5 grains.

ANGELICA

Angelica archangelica; part used: the root and the seeds

(German: *Engelwurzel*   French: *Angélique*   Spanish: *Angélica*)

This very useful aromatic stimulant relieves gas and colicky pains in the stomach and congestion in the abdomen. Its nerve-quieting effect also deserves mentioning.

Recent Findings: Test-tube and culture studies of angelica and related species have shown that the root is active in destroying fungi, as an anti-inflammatory agent and a smooth muscle relaxant, and as both a uterine stimulant and relaxant. Animal studies in China and Japan using root preparations of various *Angelica* species have shown pain-killing properties, uterine-stimulant effects, diuretic and abortifacient activity, and the ability to lower blood pressure. In humans, root preparations of *Angelica* species have been found effective in treating hemorrhoids and have demonstrated central nervous system effects adapted to use against the symptoms of polio.

Dose: 30–60 grains.

ANISE

Pimpinella anisum; part used: the seeds

(German: *Anis Samen*   French: *Anis vert*   Spanish: *Anis*)

A decoction of anise seeds added to milk relieves gas pains and colic in small children. It has a very quieting and soothing effect. Used by the nursing mother, it increases the milk secretion and stimulates the action of the stomach. It is also extensively used as a flavoring agent in pastries, etc.

Recent Findings: Anise seeds have been shown to possess insecticidal properties.

Average dose: 30 grains.

ARNICA

Arnica montana; part used: the flowers

(German: *Arnicablüten*   French: *Fleurs d'Arnique*   Spanish: *Flor de Arnica*)

In the United States, arnica has mostly been used in the form of the tincture as an external application for sprains and bruises, to relieve inflammation and swelling. In Europe, however, it is also used internally in the treatment of gout, rheumatism, and feverish conditions.

Recent Findings: Animal and human studies have verified the actions claimed for arnica, but the chemical constituents responsible have not been identified.

Dose: 5–10 grains, three or four times a day.

BETH ROOT

Trillium erectum; part used: the root

A highly prized native American remedy to stop bleeding from the lungs, bowels, kidneys, and to arrest excessive menstrual flow. In coughs, bronchitis, and asthmatic conditions, it is said to give quick and certain relief.

Recent Findings: In experiments with the root extract of *Trillium* species related to beth root, Japanese researchers demonstrated anti-ulcer activity in the rat.

Average dose: 30 grains.

BLACKBERRY

Rubus villosus; part used: the bark of the root

(German: *Brombeer Rinde*   French: *Écorce de Ronce Noir* Spanish: *Zanzamora*)

This is an excellent remedy for diarrhea, dysentery, summer complaints in children, and loose conditions of stomach and bowels. A decoction of the bark is used as a douche in leukorrhea and in relaxed conditions of the uterus.

Recent Findings: Preparations of *Rubus* species have been shown to have both uterine-stimulant and uterine-relaxant effects in test-tube studies, as well as antiviral activity against a variety of virus cultures. In animal studies, *Rubus* preparations have shown central

194

nervous system stimulant properties as well as weak depressant effects in the mouse, uterine-relaxant effects in the cat, and uterine-stimulant effects in the rabbit. *Rubus* preparations have also been shown to lower blood pressure in the dog, to act as a diuretic in the rat, to reduce temperature in the mouse, and to act as an anti-inflammatory agent in the rat.

Dose: 15–30 grains.

BLACK BIRCH

Betula lenta; part used: the leaves
(German: *Birke*   French: *Bouleau*   Spanish: *Abedul*)

Useful in looseness of the bowels in adults and children, and for producing sweating, if used warm as a tea. It has also been highly recommended in complaints of the urinary organs, inflammation or gravel in kidneys and bladder.

Recent Findings: Test-tube and culture studies have shown preparations of black birch and related species to have antifungal properties, and strong uterine-stimulant activity.

Dose: 60 grains.

BLACK COHOSH

Cimicifuga racemosa; part used: the root
(German: *Schwarze Schlangenwurzel*   French: *Racine d'Actée à Grappes*)

This root is particularly useful in rheumatic affections and in uterine disorders. In menstrual cramps, leukorrhea, and irregular menses it is invaluable. It also has a quieting and strengthening effect on the nervous system, soothing pain and relieving fever and inflammation.

Recent Findings: Root extracts of black cohosh have been shown to reduce experimental inflammation in animal studies; this provides a basis for the traditional use of this plant in neuralgia and rheumatism. Although black cohosh has traditionally been used in female complaints as well, extracts have not been shown to produce an estrogenic effect in mice; the folk use of black cohosh for menstrual problems is therefore probably not owing to an estrogenic effect.

Average dose: 15 grains.

BLOOD ROOT

Sanguinaria canadensis; part used: the root
(German: *Blutwurzel*   French: *Sanguinaire*)

This root is a very active stimulating agent and should be used carefully. In small doses, from ½ to 5 grains, it is an effective expectorant; up to 20 grains it acts as an emetic and may be used in cases where a quick emptying of the stomach is desired. Applied externally as a powder to skin eruptions, nose polyps, ulcers, and badly healing sores, it exerts great healing power, encouraging new and healthy tissue.

Recent Findings: Blood root preparations have been shown experimentally to have emetic, expectorant, and irritant properties, all owing to the toxic alkaloid *sanguinarine.* The use of sanguinarine and blood root in skin conditions is probably based on their local anesthetic properties.

Average dose: 2 grains.

BONESET

Eupatorium perfoliatum; part used: the entire plant
(German: *Wasserdost*   French: *Eupatore perfoilée*)

Its fever-reducing and sweat-inducing properties make this plant one of the most valuable herbs in colds and fevers. Catarrhal conditions due to colds yield quickly to the healing effect of this wonderful plant. It is also highly recommended as a cold preventive.

Recent Findings: The leaves of boneset contain *sesquiterpene lactones,* which act as appetite stimulants; in large enough doses, these substances help expel intestinal worms.

Average dose: 30 grains.

BROOM

Cytisus scoparius; part used: the dried tops
(German: *Besenginster*   French: *Genet à balais*   Spanish: *Retama*)

This remedy is highly recommended in disorders of the urinary organs, especially in such cases where the urine is retained or flows

196

scantily or painfully. It increases the flow of urine in dropsical conditions (swelling due to fluid retention), and relieves spasms in the bladder. It also has a tonic effect on the heart.

Average dose: 15 grains.

BUCHU

Agathosma crenulata and var. spp.; part used: the leaves
(German: *Buckublätter*   French: *Feuilles de Bucco*)

This is one of the best and most useful herbs in urinary tract diseases that are attended with increased uric acid. It relieves catarrhal conditions and inflammation in the kidneys and cramps in the bladder. It has also been recommended for gravel and stones in kidneys and bladder. Its soothing and strengthening effect on the urinary organs is highly praised.

Dose: 30 grains.

BUCKBEAN

Menyanthes trifoliata; part used: the leaves
(German: *Bitterklee*   French: *Trefle d'eau*   Spanish: *Trébol*)

This is an excellent remedy for improving the quality and flow of the digestive juices. It exerts a good influence on stomach and bowels, relieving gas and excess acid in these organs. Its prompt action in fever and colds makes it a valued and well-known botanical.

Recent Findings: The leaves contain a number of alkaloids, among which *gentianine* has been shown to have pain-killing and tranquilizing effects in animals, and *gentianadine* to reduce blood pressure and decrease inflammation.

Dose: 30 grains.

BUCKTHORN

Rhamnus cathartica, R. frangula; part used: the bark; the berries
(German: *Faulbaum Rinde*   French: *Écorce de Bourdaine*
Spanish: *Arraclan*)

This bark, like the American variety, cascara sagrada bark, should be at least two years old before it is used; it then acts as a mild yet reliable and effective laxative, stimulating the action of stomach and bowels very favorably. If used fresh, it may cause considerable griping pain and vomiting.

Recent Findings: The berries of *Rhamnus cathartica* contain *anthraquinone glycosides,* which account for the cathartic effect of the fruit of this species. The bark of *R. frangula,* widely used in Europe as a cathartic, contains the same active principles as *R. purshiana,* or cascara sagrada; these constituents are discussed under the latter plant below.

Average dose: 15–30 grains.

BURDOCK
Arctium lappa; part used: the root and the seeds
(German: *Klettenwurzel* French: *Bardane* Spanish: *Lampazo*)
This root is known for its blood-cleansing properties and is therefore used in innumerable spring medicines and blood remedies. Skin eruptions, due to impurities in the blood, yield quickly to its cleansing properties. It is extensively used in lymphatic, liver, rheumatic, and skin diseases. The seeds are used in disorders of the kidneys. Burdock oil has been very highly recommended as an external application to the scalp, to stop the falling out of hair.

Recent Findings: In animal experiments, burdock root extracts have been shown to promote urination and to inhibit tumors, to lower blood sugar, and to have estrogenic activity. Burdock extracts have been shown to destroy bacteria and fungus cultures. These experiments provide a basis for using burdock in treating diabetes, female complaints, and bacterial or fungal infections.

Average dose: Of the root or seeds, 30 grains.

CASCARA SAGRADA
Rhamnus purshiana; part used: the bark
(German: *Cascara Rinde* French: *Écorce Sagrada* Spanish:
Cascara Sagrada)
This is one of the most useful among the popular botanical laxatives. Its mild and yet effective action on the bowels makes it a favorite with many. It acts by increasing the muscular action of the intestines, toning and cleansing them. It is especially valuable in the treatment

of cases of longer standing. It should be at least two years old before it is used.

Recent Findings: Cascara contains a mixture of anthraquinones, which irritate the intestinal wall, causing catharsis; in the form of sugar derivatives *(glycosides),* they are absorbed from the intestine and carried by the bloodstream to a nerve center in the lower intestine, where they cause a laxative effect.

Dose: 15–30 grains.

CENTAURY
Chironia centaurium; part used: the flowering herb
(German: *Tausendguldenkraut* French: *Petite centaurée*
Spanish: *Centaura menor*)

This herb enjoys great popularity in Europe as a remedy for stomach disorders. It increases the appetite and invigorates the digestion. It is especially effective in cases where a tonic and blood builder is required on account of poor function of the digestive organs.

Recent Findings: Bulgarian researchers found centaury alcohol extracts to have anticonvulsant properties when administered to mice.

Average dose: 30 grains.

CHAMOMILE (GERMAN)
Matricaria chamomilla; part used: the flowers
(German: *Kamillen* French: *Camomille* Spanish: *Manzanilla*)

This is one of the oldest and most popular remedies for gas and cramps in the stomach. Its soothing, pain-relieving effects in stomach disorders and menstrual irregularities make it a most valued medicinal agent, especially in cases where these troubles are of a nervous origin. The infusion is used externally with good results in compresses to relieve pain and swelling. It has also been extensively used as a hairwash to brighten the hair.

Recent Findings: In a study with heart disease patients, chamomile tea induced sleep within ten minutes after drinking the tea; there was also a small increase in blood pressure. In animal experiments, the oil from chamomile flowers reduced elevated blood-urea levels in rabbits with impaired kidney function. Another animal experiment showed that a chemical constituent in chamomile flowers acted as an antihistamine; and chamomile essential oil reduced experimental arthritic inflammation in rats. In test tubes, chamomile oil has been shown to relax the smooth muscle of the intestine.

Dose: 30–60 grains.

CHICORY
Cichorium intybus; part used: the root and leaves
(German: *Wegwart*   French: *Chicorée*   Spanish: *Achicoria amarga*)

The root is very useful as a tonic and mild laxative. In congestion of the liver, jaundice, and other obstructions of the internal organs, it has proven very beneficial. The roasted root is used extensively as a coffee substitute. The leaves have similar properties.

Recent Findings: In test-tube studies, chicory leaf has been shown to possess uterine-relaxant properties, and the root to act as a myocardial depressant. Leaf preparations have shown weak activity against tubercle bacillus cultures. Animal studies have borne out the plant's properties of stimulating bile and combating liver toxicity in rat and mouse tests; other workers have shown abortifacient and anti-inflammatory activity in the rat, and the lowering of blood pressure in rabbits. Italian researchers found laxative properties in chicory root extract when administered to humans.

Dose: Of root or leaves, 60–120 grains.

CINCHONA
Cinchona pubescens and var. spp.; part used: the bark
(German: *China Rinde*   French: *Écorce de Quinquina*   Spanish: *Quina*)

This is a very effective remedy for general weakness due to impaired digestion and incomplete assimilation of the food. It acts as an antiseptic and astringent tonic on stomach and bowels, aids the digestion, and relieves gas and excess acid resulting from faulty digestion.

It has proven to be one of the most useful fever and cold remedies known. It is also said to have a pronounced action on the nervous system and has therefore been considered very useful in nervous dyspepsia and hysteria. Externally in the form of a poultice it is a valuable remedy for slow-healing ulcers and old, open sores.

Recent Findings: The alkaloid *quinine,* derived from cinchona bark, has long been recognized for its antimalarial properties. Overdoses of cinchona can lead to buzzing in the ears, headache, nausea, and vertigo; when ringing in the ears occurs, it is a warning that the dose should be reduced. More recently, quinine has been found to be an effective treatment for a new strain of malarial parasite that developed during the Vietnam war and was resistant to other antimalarial drugs, including the new synthetics.

Dose: 10–60 grains.

COLTSFOOT

Tussilago farfara; part used: the leaves
(German: *Huflattich*   French: *Pas d'âne*   Spanish: *Una de caballo*)

This herb is very useful in affections of the bronchial tubes and lungs. It facilitates the loosening of phlegm, and relieves cough and colds that have settled in the air passages.

Recent Findings: Test-tube and culture studies have shown coltsfoot extracts to have anti-inflammatory, antispasmodic, and antituberculous properties. Coltsfoot leaves, in a mixture with other plants, when smoked by human subjects, had antiasthmatic activity, but it is not known whether it was the coltsfoot or other plants in the mixture that accounted for these results. In animal studies in China, coltsfoot flowers, when added to the diet, were observed to be strongly active in producing liver tumors in rats; because of this finding, coltsfoot should probably not be used internally until further research has been done on its possible carcinogenic properties.

Dose: Not recommended. Average dose was generally 60 grains.

COMFREY

Symphytum officinale; part used: the root
(German: *Beinwell*   French: *Consoude*   Spanish: *Consuelda major*)

This root is very useful in lung ailments, coughs, and colds in lungs and throat. It relieves inflammation of the air passages and loosens and removes phlegm.

Recent Findings: Recent studies have shown that comfrey contains potentially toxic and/or carcinogenic substances; for this reason, it should not be used internally until the issue of its toxicity has been resolved. With this caution in mind, it is probably safe to use comfrey leaves as an external application, to promote healing of wounds and broken bones.

Dose: Not recommended for internal use. Dose was formerly 30–60 grains.

COUCH GRASS

Agropyron repens; part used: the root and rhizome
(German: *Queckenwurzel*   French: *Chiendent*   Spanish: *Rizoma de Grama*)

Couch grass is very valuable in disorders of kidneys and bladder and in urinary troubles that originate with colds or catarrhal inflammation of these organs. It induces the proper flow of the urine and tends to relieve painful, scanty but frequent urination. Its blood-purifying properties are also quite pronounced.

Recent Findings: The roots of couch grass contain mucilage, which accounts for the plant's soothing and demulcent action on mucous membranes. Animal studies in Rumania showed that couch grass rhizome preparations had a diuretic effect in rats, and workers in Tanganyika found strong central nervous system depressant activity in mice. Extracts have also been shown to have antibiotic effects against bacteria and molds.

Average dose: 60–120 grains.

CRAMP BARK

Viburnum opulus; part used: the bark
(German: *Schneeball Rinde*   French: *Obier*)

As its name indicates, this bark is very effective in relieving cramps and spasms of all kinds. As it also exerts a decided influence upon the reproductive organs, it is especially useful in menstrual cramps and pains, giving tone and energy to the uterus. It is claimed that its use during pregnancy tends to diminish miscarriage, especially if used with equal parts of button snakeroot.

Recent Findings: Test-tube studies have shown cramp bark to be active as a smooth muscle relaxant, a cardiotonic, and to have both uterine-stimulant and uterine-relaxant properties. Preparations of a related species, *V. prunifolium,* have been shown to produce abortion and to stimulate gastric secretions in humans. Animal studies have additionally shown *Viburnum* species extracts to reduce blood pressure in the dog and to lower body temperature in the mouse.

Average dose: 30 grains.

DANDELION

Taraxacum officinale; part used: the root and the leaves
(German: *Löwenzahn*   French: *Dent de Lion, Pissenlit*
Spanish: *Diente de Leon*)

The blood-cleansing properties of this simple root, and its stimulating effect on stomach, liver, and bowels, make it a very valuable botanical for all disorders of these organs.

The leaves used fresh as a salad invigorate the functions of the digestive organs; they are rich in iron and other valuable mineral elements. In the event the fresh leaves cannot be obtained, the dried leaves will do.

Recent Findings: Dandelion root extracts have been shown to increase secretion of bile in laboratory animals, which might account for the use of dandelion in liver disorders. Although the active principle responsible for this effect has not been identified, the roots are known to contain *inulin,* an essential oil and a bitter compound.

Average dose: 60–120 grains.

DOG ROSE

Rosa canina; part used: the fruit
(German: *Hagebutton*   French: *Gratte cul*   Spanish: *Calambrujo cirosbatos*)

This fruit is rich in citric and malic acids and is said to have wonderful dissolving properties on stones of kidneys and bladder.

Recent Findings: Bulgarian studies showed the essential oil from the flowers of dog rose to have antihistaminic, antispasmodic, laxative, and bile-stimulating effects in humans. Animal studies with extracts of related species have demonstrated anti-tumor and anti-inflammatory activity in the rat, central nervous system depressant effects in the mouse, lowering of blood pressure in the cat, and diuretic activity in the rat. Test-tube and culture studies have revealed antiviral, uterine-stimulant, and spasm-relieving effects for preparations of various species of *Rosa*.

Dose: 60 grains.

DWARF ELDER

Sambucus ebulus; part used: the root
(German: *Attich Wurzel*   French: *Hièble*   Spanish: *Yezgo*)
This root is a valued remedy for disorders of kidneys and bladder; especially in dropsical conditions (swelling due to fluid retention) it is said to give good results.

Recent Findings: See ELDER.

Dose: 15–30 grains.

DWARF NETTLE

Urtica urens; part used: the entire green plant and the root
(German: *Brenn-Nessel*   French: *Ortie*   Spanish: *Ortiga*)
This plant is rich in organic mineral substances and therefore valuable as a blood and system cleanser. Because of its diuretic properties, it reduces the acid content of the blood and eliminates impurities through the kidneys and bladder. it can be used with good results in looseness or bleeding of the bowels.

A decoction or extraction of the root used on the scalp is a most favored remedy in Europe for falling hair.

Dose: 30–60 grains.

ELDER

Sambucus canadensis, S. nigra; part used: the flowers, the berries, the root

(German: *Hollunder Blüten*   French: *Fleur de Sureau*   Spanish: *Sauco*)

The flowers made into a tea open the pores and produce sweating. In that manner they aid in eliminating acids and other impurities through the skin. They are, therefore, very valuable in the treatment of colds, coughs, and rheumatic and catarrhal conditions associated with suppressed skin action.

Recent Findings: Elder-leaf extract has been shown to have antiviral activity in virus-culture studies.

Average dose: 60 grains.

ELECAMPANE

Inula helenium; part used: the root

(German: *Alant*   French: *Aunée*   Spanish: *Enula Campana*)

This is a very useful remedy for coughs and colds in bronchial tubes and lungs. It assists in loosening phlegm and relieves irritation in the air passages.

Average dose: 30 grains.

EYEBRIGHT

Euphrasia officinalis; part used: the plant

(German: *Augentrost*   French: *Euphrasie*   Spanish: *Eufrasia*)

An infusion of one part of this herb to six parts of water has been found to be very beneficial when applied to the eyes and eyelids in catarrhal and inflamed conditions of the eyes; it exerts a soothing, healing, and strengthening action.

Dose: 60 grains.

FENNEL

Foeniculum vulgare; part used: the seed

(German: *Fenchel*   French: *Fenouil*   Spanish: *Hinojo*)

In gas colic and spasms in children, fennel tea (one teaspoonful of the seeds to a cup of water or milk) is one of the best and safest remedies. Made into a syrup with the addition of honey or sugar, it relieves coughs and colds.

Preparations of fennel water, available in apothecary shops, have been a highly valued remedy in Europe for tired, sore eyes. Fennel seeds should be on hand in every household.

Recent Findings: Fennel oil has been shown to have antifungal activity in cell culture studies, and to have antispasmodic properties in test-tube experiments. In animal studies, the fruit has been shown to be effective as an insect repellent, and the essential oil to have estrogenic effects in mice and rats and to act as a central nervous system depressant in mice and goldfish.

Average dose: 15–30 grains.

FLAX SEED

Linum usitatissimum; part used: the seed

(German: *Leinsamen*   French: *Grains de lin*   Spanish: *Lino*)

An infusion of these seeds is very useful in catarrhal conditions of the bronchial tubes and also of the urinary organs. In disorders of kidneys and bladder, it may be used freely; its action is very soothing and healing. Ground flax seed, mixed with hot water to form a stiff paste, makes an excellent emollient poultice for local inflammations, boils, and carbuncles. The whole seed is also occasionally given in table-spoonful doses as a mild laxative.

Dose: 60–120 grains.

GENTIAN (YELLOW)

Gentiana lutea; part used: the root

(German: *Enzian*   French: *Gentiane*   Spanish: *Genciana*)

This is a great and much valued remedy in all cases where a stomach tonic is required. It incites the appetite, invigorates digestion, relieves gases, and reduces excessive amounts of acid produced by faulty digestion. The chewing of this root aids in overcoming the desire for the chewing and smoking of tobacco.

Average dose: 15 grains.

GINGER
Zingiber officinale; part used: the root

This aromatic root acts as a stimulating tonic on the stomach, increasing the secretions of the gastric juices and dispelling gases from stomach and bowels. It is useful for abdominal cramps and pains; in looseness of the bowels and in diarrhea and dysentery, it produces excellent results, especially when combined with other astringents, such as oak bark, alum root, etc.

Recent Findings: In test-tube experiments, ginger rhizome preparations have been observed to have anticonvulsant and antispasmodic activity, while Indian researchers have found ginger to have anticholesterol activity in the rat.

Average dose: 10 grains.

GOLDEN SEAL
Hydrastis canadensis; part used: the root
(German: *Kanadische Gelbwurzel*   French: *Racine d'Hydrastis du Canada*   Spanish: *Hidrastis del Canada*)

The tonic properties of this root are remarkable, and its healing and strengthening influence on the mucous membrane and muscular tissues make it a very valuable remedy in catarrhal inflammations of the mucous membrane. It is, therefore, very valuable in catarrh of stomach and bowels. Externally it is used in catarrh of the head and throat, and in vaginal catarrh. The decoction can be used as an eyewash with good results. Its pain-relieving and soothing properties also deserve mentioning.

Recent Findings: External applications of golden seal to the arms and legs have been shown to relieve disorders of the blood vessels and lymphatics. The alkaloid *berberine,* a constituent of golden seal, has been shown to have anticonvulsive effects on the intestines and uterus, and to destroy *Staphylococcus aureus* bacteria.

Average dose: 30 grains.

GROUND IVY

Glechoma hederacea; part used: the plant
(German: *Gundelrebe*   French: *Lierre terrestre*   Spanish: *Hiedra*)
This herb is especially useful in catarrhal inflammations of the inner organs—lungs, stomach, bowels, and the urinary tract.
Dose: 30–60 grains.

HOREHOUND

Marrubium vulgare; part used: the herb
(German: *Weisser Andorn*   French: *Marrube blanc*   Spanish: *Marrubio*)
A valuable expectorant. It is used in affections of throat and lungs.
Recent Findings: The high concentration of mucilage in horehound accounts for its soothing effect on sore throats. The other uses of the plant have thus far not been supported by experimental evidence.
Dose: 30–60 grains.

JUNIPER

Juniperus communis; part used: the berries
(German: *Wacholderbeeren*   French: *Baies de Genièvre*
Spanish: *Bayas de Enebro*)
These berries are highly recommended in catarrhal conditions of the urinary organs, in rheumatism, gout, and fluid retention. In small doses, they incite the appetite and aid the digestion, but in larger doses they act more on the kidneys and bladder.
Recent Findings: Juniper berries have been shown experimentally to have anti-tumor activity in animals. The diuretic effect of the berries has been demonstrated in animals. Studies on humans have shown that the berries have value in treating arthritis, substantiating the traditional use of the plant in inflammatory conditions. The mildly stimulant effect of the berries is attributed to the constituents of the essential oil.
Dose: 60 grains.

Materia Medica

KNOT GRASS

Polygonum aviculare; part used: the plant

(German: *Knöterich*   French: *Centinode*   Spanish: *Centinoda*)

This insignificant-looking, plain little plant possesses wonderful properties and is one of the most effective remedies in affections of the bronchial tubes and lungs. Its soothing and healing effect on these organs is remarkable; it relieves coughs, loosens the phlegm, allays irritation and tickling in the throat.

It is also of great value in the treatment of gravel and stones of kidneys and bladder.

Recent Findings: South Korean workers have demonstrated anti-inflammatory properties for knot grass in test-tube studies, while test-tube and culture studies showed preparations of other *Polygonum* species to be weakly active against tubercle bacillus, to be active in semen coagulation (suggesting possible contraceptive applications), to have antispasmodic properties, and to have active to strongly active uterine stimulant properties as well as active uterine relaxant properties.

Extracts of various *Polygonum* species have been shown in animal experiments to reduce blood pressure in the rabbit, reduce blood sugar in the dog, decrease temperature in the mouse, exhibit anti-tumor activity in the rat, act as a central nervous system depressant in the mouse, have hemostatic properties in the mouse and the guinea pig, and have anti-inflammatory properties and accelerate the healing of burns in the rat. One species, *P. hydropiper,* was shown in English experiments to suppress the production of sperm and of gonadotropins and estrogens when added to the diet of the mouse, while root extracts of the same species were found by researchers in India to have embryotoxic and anti-implantation effects in the rat. All these findings would suggest that *Polygonum* species may be of value in birth control.

Knot grass was included in a mixture that facilitated ureteral stone removal in humans in a Chinese study, but because several other plants were involved, it is not known whether this action was attributable to this plant. Preparations of other *Polygonum* species have been effective in humans as a local anesthetic for tooth pain and as a hemostatic against hemorrhage and excessive menstrual bleeding.

Dose: 30–60 grains.

LICORICE

Glycyrrhiza glabra; part used: the root
(German: *Süssholz*   French: *Réglisse*   Spanish: *Crozuz*)

This very useful expectorant is used in coughs and bronchial irritations. It is extensively used as a sweetening agent for diet drinks and bitter medicines. It is also mildly laxative.

Recent Findings: The effects of licorice rhizomes and roots are largely due to the compound *glycyrrhizin,* which is about fifty times sweeter than sugar and produces a cortisone-like effect that can lead to toxic symptoms in overdose. The rhizomes and roots also have a high mucilage content; when mixed with water, the root therefore makes a very pleasant-smelling and -tasting preparation for soothing irritated mucous membranes.

Dose: 30 grains.

LINDEN

Tilia europaea; part used: the flowers
(German: *Lindenblüten*   French: *Tilleul*   Spanish: *Tilo*)

These sweet, honey-scented flowers are excellent for loosening the phlegm from bronchial tubes and stomach. They also tend to quiet the nerves and relieve cramps. The warm infusion acts as a mild sweat-producer. The flowers are used extensively in colds and coughs. In many parts of Europe they are used in place of ordinary tea. They make a palatable after-meal beverage, with the added advantage of having a soothing effect upon the nerves and aiding digestion.

Recent Findings: Indian workers have shown linden extracts to be effective against virus cultures; preparations of other *Tilia* species have exhibited estrogenic and anticonvulsant activity in the mouse.

Dose: 60 grains.

LUNGWORT

Pulmonaria officinalis; part used: the herb
(German: *Lungenkraut*   French: *Pulmonaire*   Spanish:
Pulmonaria)

As its name indicates, lungwort has been found valuable in the treatment of affections of the lungs and air passages. It relieves inflamed conditions and is used in coughs and colds.

Dose: 30 grains.

MALLOW

Malva sylvestris: part used: the leaves
(German: *Malva*   French: *Mauve*   Spanish: *Malva real*)

This is a useful remedy for coughs and colds and for obstructed breathing caused by phlegm in the air passages. It is also used externally in the form of poultices and fomentations for the relief of inflammation and pain; they are very healing and soothing when applied to open sores and ulcers.

Recent Findings: South Korean workers found mallow seed extract to have anti-inflammatory activity in test-tube studies, while Japanese experiments showed a leaf and stem extract of a related species to have a stimulant effect on uterine tissue.

Dose: 30 grains.

MANDRAKE

Podophyllum peltatum; part used: the root
(German: *Podophyll Wurzel*   French: *Rhizone de Podophyllum*
Spanish: *Podofilo*)

For liver and bowel complaints this American root has proven equal, if not superior, to its more expensive foreign counterparts. It is a valuable aid in biliousness, constipation, and other disturbances due to sluggish action of liver and bowels. Its eliminative properties make it very effective as well in rheumatism and other diseases marked by an accumulation of waste products in the system. As an expeller of intestinal worms, it is also highly recommended.

Dose: 10–30 grains.

Caution: An overdose would likely be fatal. Pregnant women must

211

not take any remedy containing this herb, which may cause birth defects.

MARSH MALLOW
Althaea officinalis; part used: the root
(German: *Eibisch Wurzel*   French: *Racine de Guimauve*
Spanish: *Raiz de Malvavisco*)

This valuable demulcent is used in inflammation and irritation of the mucous membrane. It is recommended in coughs and complaints of the bronchial tubes, and in disorders of the kidneys and bladder.

Dose: 30–60 grains.

MATÉ
Ilex paraguayensis; part used: the leaves

From this South American plant, a delightfully refreshing drink is made that is justly called "South America's national beverage." Its stimulating and invigorating effect on the body, and its quieting and strengthening effect on the nervous system, make it the ideal substitute for ordinary tea or coffee. On account of its low tannin content, which amounts to only 1 to 2 percent, it is not constipating like ordinary tea with its 13 to 18 percent tannin (tannin is very constipating). Its richness in natural mineral salts—calcium, magnesium, iron, manganese, silica, phosphates—as well as vitamins, adds greatly to its usefulness as a beverage.

It is prepared like ordinary tea—about a teaspoonful to a cup of boiling water. Sugar, honey, cream, and lemon may be added to suit taste. When iced, it makes a refreshing summer drink.

Recent Findings: Reports of toxic effects from ingestion of maté leaf and fruit preparations by humans must be considered questionable, since the identity of the plant is not well established in these cases. Preparations of related *Ilex* species have been shown to have emollient and central nervous system depressant effects in humans, and Chinese workers successfully used the leaf extract of an *Ilex* species as a postoperative medication to dilate blood vessels following limb reimplantations.

Dose: 60 grains.

MISTLETOE

Viscum album; part used: the plant
(German: *Mistel*   French: *Gui de chêne*   Spanish: *Muérdago*)
This plant has proved of service in high blood pressure and in stopping excessive menstrual flow. It tends to relieve spasms and pains encountered during the menstrual period.

Recent Findings: Experiments with both animals and humans have shown that mistletoe preparations have sedative properties. Although there have been reports that animals and children have been poisoned by mistletoe berries, there is no documentation of such adverse effects. Mistletoe, however, does contain *tyramine*, which, when taken in combination with a monoaminoxidase (MAO) inhibitor (prescription drugs that regulate blood pressure), can cause a serious drop in blood pressure. One should be careful, therefore, not to take mistletoe preparations (or certain other foods that also contain tyramine, such as aged cheeses, cured meats, and Chianti wine) at the same time one is taking an MAO inhibitor.

Dose: 15–30 grains.

MULLEIN

Verbascum thapsus; part used: the leaves and the flowers
(German: *Wollkraut*   French: *Bouillon blanc*   Spanish:
Gordolobo)
The leaves and the flowers are used in chest complaints; they possess softening, soothing, lubricating, and slightly pain-relieving properties. Mullein is given for coughs and catarrhal conditions of the throat and lungs.

Dose: 30–60 grains.

OAK (RED AND WHITE)

Quercus rubra, Q. alba; part used: the bark
(German: *Eichenrinde*   French: *Écorce de Chêne*   Spanish:
Encina Roble)
The bark of the red oak *(Q. rubra)* and the white oak *(Q. alba)* are both used medicinally. Their properties are the same and therefore both can be used for the same purpose. Oak bark possesses strong

astringent and antiseptic properties. It is used internally in diarrhea and to stop mucous discharges and bleeding. In the form of a decoction it is used as a gargle for sore throat and as an injection for leukorrhea and hemorrhoids. Poultices of the ground bark are used with good results in ulcers and badly healing sores.

The acorns of the oak are roasted like coffee and are used as a substitute for coffee or tea, especially by those who suffer from looseness of the bowels.

Dose: Of the bark, 15 grains.

OATS
Avena sativa; part used: the straw
(German: *Haferstroh*   French: *Avoine*   Spanish: *Avena*)

Oat straw has been extensively used to supply the body with the element *silicon,* in which it is very rich and which it contains in a very assimilable form. Silicon is the substance necessary to build the outer layer of the skin, the hair, the fingernails, and so on; deficiencies of silicon often cause such problems as splitting or deformed fingernails, and skin diseases

The use of the seeds as a food of great value is too well known to need mentioning here.

Recent Findings: Workers in the United States and in Israel have shown oats to have both estrogenic and antiestrogenic effects in rats and mice.

Dose: Of oat straw, 30–60 grains.

OREGON GRAPE ROOT
Berberis aquifolium; part used: the root
(German: *Berberitze, Sauerdorn*   French: *Vinettier*   Spanish: *Berbero*)

An old native American remedy of great merit, this root is very valuable in jaundice, sluggishness of the liver and bowels, and rheumatic conditions. It increases the power of the digestive organs and aids the assimilation of food. Its blood-cleansing properties make it also a much used remedy in skin diseases, scrofula, pimples, and boils.

Recent Findings: The alkaloid *berberine* accounts for most of the effects of the root. When applied externally, berberine has an astringent effect, as well as producing mild local anesthesia. Berberine can have a purgative action in larger doses, but can also be used to stop diarrhea in cases of bacterial dysentery.

Dose: 30 grains.

PANSY
Viola tricolor; part used: the herb
(German: *Stiefmütterchen*   French: *Pensée sauvage*   Spanish: *Pensamiento*)

The blood-cleansing properties of this modest little plant are hardly excelled by any other. Especially in scrofula and skin eruptions in children good results are obtained. It is rich in mineral salts and is an effective purgative and liver regulator.

Average dose: 15–30 grains.

PENNYROYAL
Hedeoma pulegioides; part used: the herb
(German: *Polei amerikanischer*   French: *Poulist Américaine*)

This gentle aromatic stimulant is used especially in flatulent colic and stomach disorders due to fermentation of the food. It stimulates the menstrual flow and tends to relieve cramps due to suppressed menstruation. A warm infusion produces sweating and has been found of good service in colds.

Recent Findings: Pennyroyal extracts have been shown to stimulate uterine tissue in test-tube experiments, which may account for the plant's ability to promote menstruation. Large doses of the plant have been shown to produce nausea, vomiting, and possible toxicity.

Average dose: 60 grains.

PEPPERMINT
Mentha piperita; part used: the leaves
(German: *Pfefferminze*   French: *Menthe poivrée*   Spanish: *Menta piperita*)

The strengthening and refreshing effect that this herb has on the digestive organs is well recognized. Taken in the form of an infusion, it aids digestion and relieves gas and spasms. Its beneficial influence on the nervous system and heart also deserves mentioning.

Recent Findings: The effects of the plant have been shown in animal experiments to be due to the constituents of the essential oil.

Dose: 60 grains.

PINK ROOT
Spigelia marilandica; part used: the root
(German: *Wurmgrass Wurzel* French: *Spigélie anthelminthique*)

This is an excellent worm expeller; it removes stomach and intestinal worms quickly, but is best used in combination with cathartics in correct dosages. An overdose may cause unpleasant contributory symptoms.

Dose: For a child, 10–20 grains; for an adult, 1–2 drachms (60–120 grains), either in powder form or as a tea.

PIPSISSEWA
Chimaphila umbellata; part used: the leaves

These leaves are extensively used in disorders of the urinary organs, especially to relieve irritation and catarrhal conditions of kidneys and bladder, to reduce uric acid, and against deposits of stones and gravel.

Recent Findings: The leaves contain the chemicals *ericolin, arbutin, chimaphilin, urson, tannin,* and *gallic acid.* Chimaphilin, as well as plant extracts, has been shown to have antibacterial properties in test-tube experiments.

Dose: 30 grains.

PLANTAIN
Plantago officinalis and var. spp.; part used: the leaves
(German: *Wegerich* French: *Plantain* Spanish: *Llanten*)

This valuable expectorant relieves coughs, bronchitis, and hoarseness, and loosens catarrhal obstructions from bronchial tubes and lungs. It is also used externally as a poultice on old, badly healing ulcers and sores, inflamed eyes and muscles.

Recent Findings: Preparations of various *Plantago* species have shown antiviral and antibacterial activity when used to treat culture preparations, and test-tube studies have shown anti-inflammatory properties. Researchers in India and the USSR have demonstrated the ability of *Plantago* preparations to lower blood cholesterol levels in the rabbit. In humans, *Plantago*-seed preparations have been shown to have a laxative effect, and Chinese workers have demonstrated the efficacy of seed extracts in removing ureteral stones.

Average dose: 60 grains.

PLEURISY ROOT
Asclepias tuberosa; part used: the root
(German: *Schwalben Wurzel* French: *Racine d'Asclépiade tubereuse*)

As its name indicates, this is a very valuable remedy for pleurisy, catarrhal affections of the lungs and throat, and spasmodic coughs. It is also a mild laxative and has a very beneficial effect on some forms of indigestion.

Recent Findings: The active principles responsible for the effects of this plant have not been identified.

Dose: 20–30 grains.

POKE ROOT
Phytolacca americana; part used: the root
(German: *Kermeswurzel* French: *Racine de Phytolaque*)

This root has a very favorable influence on the glandular system, inciting and increasing its action. It regulates liver and bowels and cleanses the blood. It is therefore highly valued in rheumatic conditions and skin problems due to impurities in the blood.

Recent Findings: Extracts of poke have been shown to possess activity against virus and bacteria cultures. The berries acted as a spermicide against human sperm in test-tube studies. In animal experiments, the berry has been shown to act as a central nervous system depressant, a respiratory depressant, and an agent for reducing blood pressure. In other animal studies, the root was found by South Korean workers to have anti-inflammatory activity, and American experimenters found the leaf to have laxative effects. In American studies in which varying proportions of poke berry were added to the diet of turkeys, significant weight loss resulted, which tends to bear out the folkloric claims for the plant as a reducing aid; however, at high doses there was also increased mortality. The berry of a related species, *P. dodecandra,* was found in American studies to be toxic to the rat embryo, and to induce abortion. Leaf preparations were found to be effective as a laxative in humans, and the root was shown to reduce inflammation in 53 percent of arthritic patients studied, with some reported side effects of nausea. Other human studies have yielded evidence of toxic effects including stomach cramps, diarrhea, nausea, and vomiting. *Phytolacca* preparations should therefore be used with caution.

Average dose: 1–5 grains of the dried herb only. See caution below. In large doses (10–30 grains), it acts as an emetic.

Caution: The *fresh* herb, or when insufficiently dried, is poisonous. The seeds in the berries are also toxic, particularly for children.

POMEGRANATE
Punica granatum; part used: the bark of the root
(German: *Granat Rinde*   French: *Écorce de Granadier*   Spanish: *Corteza de Granada*)

The astringent properties of this bark make it a valuable remedy in looseness of the bowels, diarrhea, and dysentery. Its greatest usefulness, however, is in the expulsion of tapeworms, where it acts very reliably if used properly. Two ounces of the bark to about a pint of water are boiled slowly for half an hour and strained while still warm. This decoction is taken in three divided doses at one-hour intervals, preferably in the morning on an empty stomach. It should be followed by a laxative. In stubborn cases, it may be necessary to repeat the treatment for a few days.

Dose: 1–2 ounces; see above.

PSYLLIUM
Plantago psyllium; part used: the seeds

The seeds are primarily used as an intestinal lubricant for the relief of habitual constipation and to promote a free and regular bowel movement. The mechanical action in the stomach, due to the swelling of the seeds, facilitates the grinding up of the food and promotes the free flow of gastric juice. In the intestines, the movement and passage of the contents are facilitated by the lubrication of the walls, the soft consistency that the seeds create, and the added bulk that they give. Psyllium seeds also have been found very useful as a demulcent to soothe, soften, and protect the mucous membrane in various affections, such as sore throat, ulcers of the stomach, diarrhea, dysentery, rectal congestion, and hemorrhoids.

Recent Findings: See PLANTAIN for discussion of *Plantago* species.

Dose: 1–2 two teaspoonfuls at each meal; more or less as needed.

RHUBARB
Rheum officinale; part used: the root
(German: *Rhabarber* French: *Rhubarbe* Spanish: *Ruibarbo*)

Rhubarb is a very valuable remedy. It incites the activity of stomach, liver, and bowels by increasing the flow of the digestive juices. In small doses, it makes an excellent strengthening tonic for the stomach, and in larger doses acts as a laxative. Its dual action as both laxative and astringent can be taken advantage of in diarrhea, hemorrhoids, and chronic dysentery. It is generally used in combination with other laxatives, which renders it more effective. The powder is often applied to indolent ulcers.

Recent Findings: The rhizomes and roots contain mixtures of anthraquinones, both in the free form and as sugar derivatives, or *glycosides.* The roots are also known to contain high concentrations of *tannins,* accounting for their astringent effect. The laxative effect of rhubarb taken in small doses is due to the action of the anthraquinones and their sugar derivatives; however, when larger amounts are taken, the action of the astringent tannins predominates, exerting an antidiarrheal effect. The tannins are also responsible for forming a protective coating when rhubarb preparations are applied to indolent ulcers. Caution must be exercised, however, in applying preparations containing tannin to large open wounds, as has been common in the treatment of severe burns. If enough tannin is absorbed into the bloodstream, it will have a toxic effect on the liver and kidneys. Toxicity and fatalities have been produced when a 3 to 5 percent tannic acid solution was used on burns.

Average dose: As a stomachic and laxative, 5–10 grains. Average dose as a cathartic is 20–30 grains.

ROSEMARY

Rosemarinus officinalis; part used: the leaves
(German: *Rosmarin* French: *Rosmarin* Spanish: *Romero*)
These spicy aromatic leaves are used for stomach and heart. They aid the digestion, increase the appetite, and check fermentation. Rosemary's heart-stimulating properties make it a valuable remedy in weak heart and in dropsical conditions (water retention) due to it.

Recent Findings: The essential oil has been shown active against fungus cultures, while Yugoslavian studies have found both central nervous depressant and spasm-producing effects when the essential oil was administered to goldfish.

Average dose: 30 grains.

RUE

Ruta graveolens; part used: the herb
(German: *Raute* French: *Rue* Spanish: *Ruda*)
Rue is an antispasmodic and stimulant. It tends to relieve gas and cramps due to nervous indigestion. It is very useful in nervous disturbances due to female irregularities. *It should not be taken by pregnant women.*

Recent Findings: Rue extracts have been shown in animal experiments to cause abortion, probably due to a direct stimulant effect on the uterine muscle by the alkaloid *skimmianine.* Large doses of rue extracts have been reported to cause poisoning in humans when taken to induce menstruation or abortion; in these cases of poisoning, some other chemical than skimmianine must be exerting a toxic effect. Some of the chemical constituents in rue can cause extreme sensitivity to sunlight; persons taking rue preparations should avoid overexposure to sunlight or they may be badly sunburned. Rue also causes severe dermatitis in some individuals. Because of the possible side effects, rue should not be taken for prolonged periods of time, nor in large doses.

Dose: 10–20 grains; see cautions above.

Caution: see above.

SAGE

Salvia officinalis; part used: the leaves

(German: *Salbei*   French: *Sauge*   Spanish: *Salvia*)

This is a reliable expectorant, and a very useful remedy for gas in stomach and bowels. It is especially valuable for the removal of slimy secretions from stomach, bronchial tubes, and lungs. For the prevention of exhausting night sweats, there is no better remedy than a cup of the infusion of sage before retiring. The decoction, used as a gargle and mouthwash, gives quick relief from inflammation, soreness, and ulceration of throat and mouth.

Recent Findings: Sage extracts have demonstrated anti-fever properties in the guinea pig, estrogenic activity in the mouse, and central nervous system depressant and spasm-producing effects in goldfish. Preparations of other *Salvia* species have shown vitamin E activity in the mouse, dilation of blood vessels in the rabbit, central nervous system depressant activity in the mouse, and reduction of blood pressure in the cat and the dog. Extracts of *Salvia* species have shown activity against cultures of viruses, amoebae, and fungi, while test-tube studies have yielded evidence of antispasmodic and anti-inflammatory properties.

Dose: 15–60 grains.

SAINT JOHN'SWORT

Hypericum perforatum; part used: the herb

(German: *Johanniskraut*   French: *Millepertuis*   Spanish: *Corazoncillo*)

This herb exerts a very beneficial influence on the nervous system, urinary organs, and liver. It is especially highly recommended in the bedwetting of children and in weakness of the bladder.

Recent Findings: The plant contains *hypericin,* which will produce dermatitis, severe sunburn, and possible blistering in light-skinned individuals on exposure to sunlight. For this reason, internal use of Saint-John'swort is *not* recommended in potentially susceptible individuals.

Dose: Usual dose was 60 grains. However, see the caution above concerning internal use.

Caution: See above.

SANICLE

Sanicula europaea; part used: the plant

(German: *Sanicle* French: *Sanicle* Spanish: *Sanicul*)

This remedy has been widely used in Europe to arrest internal bleeding from lungs, throat, stomach, and bowels. The decoction is used as a mouthwash and gives excellent results in sore, spongy, bleeding gums and in inflamed conditions of the mucous membrane of mouth and throat. Applied externally to wounds, cuts, bruises, open sores, and so on, it demonstrates its great cleansing and healing properties.

Dose: Internally, from 30 to 60 grains.

SARSAPARILLA

Smilax aristolochiifolia; part used: the root

(German: *Sarsaparilla* French: *Salsepareille* Spanish: *Zarzaparilla*)

This root has a great reputation as a blood purifier. In diseases of the skin, rheumatic afflictions, scrofula, and other diseases due to impurities in the system, it can be used with good results.

Recent Findings: Sarsaparilla root extracts have been observed to have anti–tubercle bacillus activity in culture studies, while preparations of related species have demonstrated antispasmodic and uterine-relaxant effects in test-tube experiments. The extract of another *Smilax* species has been shown to lower blood pressure in the dog and to stimulate urine production in the rat.

Dose: 30–60 grains.

SASSAFRAS

Sassafras albidum; part used: the bark of the root

(German: *Sassafrasrinde* French: *Écorce de Sassafras* Spanish: *Sassafras*)

The bark of the root is used as an alterative, a diaphoretic (sweat-producer), and stimulant. It is used to purify the blood in skin diseases and rheumatism. The infusion is also used both internally and externally for poison ivy and poison oak. Sassafras tea was traditionally a very popular spring tonic.

Recent Findings: The essential oil from the root bark has been shown experimentally to have antiseptic properties, which may account for some of the external uses of this herb. Sassafras teas, prepared as water extracts of the root bark, contain small quantities of a substance known as *safrole,* which has been shown experimentally to produce liver damage and liver cancer in rats to whom it was fed. For this reason, the U.S. Food and Drug Administration has prohibited the sale of safrole-containing substances, such as sassafras root bark, for use in foods and flavorings; however, sassafras root and root bark are still available and widely used in the United States. It is significant that the safrole itself does not produce cancer in animals, but rather must be converted to another substance. While this substance has been experimentally shown to be produced in rats, mice, and dogs, it has not been shown to be produced by humans who have taken safrole orally. It is possible that humans may convert safrole differently than do these other species, in which case the ban on sassafras root bark may eventually be lifted.

Dose: Prohibited and not recommended; see above. Formerly the usual dose was 30–60 grains.

SCOURING RUSH
Equisetum arvense; part used: the plant
(German: *Zinnkraut*   French: *Pribe des champs*   Spanish: *Cola de caballo*)

Its excellent diuretic properties make this plant one of the most useful remedies in diseases of kidneys and bladder. Inflammation, spasms, and catarrh of these organs are benefited by its use. It is used in disorders of the urinary tract, such as scanty, suppressed, frequent, or bloody urination, and in gravel and stones. Externally, it is used with good results in the form of poultices and fomentations in swollen and inflamed conditions.

Recent Findings: The plant contains *silica* in high concentrations, whose irritant action may account for the slight diuretic activity that has been shown experimentally for extracts of this plant.

Average dose: 30–60 grains.

SCULLCAP

Scutellaria laterifolia; part used: the herb

(German: *Helmkraut* French: *Scutellaire*)

This herb has a very beneficial influence on the nervous system, soothing and strengthening it. It is especially recommended in restlessness, nervous irritability, wakefulness, nervous weakness, convulsions, and seizures.

Recent Findings: Scullcap preparations have been shown to have a relaxant effect on uterine tissue in test-tube studies. Extracts of related species have been found effective against bacterial cultures. Animal studies have demonstrated *Scutellaria* species to have diuretic, bile-stimulating, anti-fever, and depressant activity, and to lower blood pressure. Chinese studies with the root extract of a *Scutellaria* species have demonstrated central nervous system depressant activity in humans.

Dose: 15 grains.

SENNA

Cassia senna; part used: the leaves

This is a mild and safe remedy for the regulation of the bowels. The leaves, however, should not be cooked but only steeped; otherwise, they may cause griping, crampy pains. By combining them with other mild cathartics and carminatives (gas expellers), the griping effect can, however, be modified or entirely eliminated.

Recent Findings: The leaves and pods contain complex *anthraquinones*, known as *sennosides*, which produce the laxative effect. Some laxative preparations are available that combine the sennosides with a stool softener, but these do not appear to be any more effective than the sennosides, or extracts of senna pods and leaves, alone.

Dose: 30 grains.

SHEPHERD'S PURSE

Capsella bursa-pastoris; part used: the herb
(German: *Hirtentäschel*   French: *Bourse à pasteur*   Spanish:
Bolso de pastor)

This insignificant-looking little plant, which grows so plentifully almost everywhere, has very valuable properties. Its decoction is used to arrest bleeding of all kinds, including hemorrhages of the lungs, stomach, and bowels. It is also extensively used for excessive menstrual flow.

Recent Findings: Extracts of the plant have been shown to prevent the formation of stress-induced duodenal ulcers in rats, and to have marked anti-inflammatory activity in other animal studies. Extracts have also demonstrated significant activity against tumors induced experimentally in laboratory animals. Animal and human studies have also shown the plant to arrest bleeding.

Dose: 15–30 grains.

SLIPPERY ELM

Ulmus fulva; part used: the inner bark
(German: *Ulmenrinde*   French: *Écorce d'Orme (fauve)*)

This is a splendid remedy for the relief of inflamed conditions of stomach and bowels, and is very beneficial in diarrhea and dysentery. It is a mild and harmless laxative for children, operating without pain. The powdered bark is an excellent emollient poultice, relieving pain and inflammation and promoting pus formation in boils and ulcers; it promotes healing in fresh wounds, bruises, burns, and swelling. The addition of equal parts of powdered fenugreek adds greatly to the efficacy of the poultice.

Dose: 60 grains.

SPEEDWELL

Veronica officinalis; part used: the herb
(German: *Ehrenpreis*   French: *Véronique*   Spanish: *Verónica*)

This herb is used in chest, kidney, and skin disorders. It cleanses the blood and tones the system.

Recent Findings: Studies on the mouse in the Soviet Union have shown a speedwell plant preparation to have central nervous system depressant activity.

Dose: 30–60 grains.

STRAWBERRY
Fragaria vesca; part used: the leaves
(German: *Erdbeere*   French: *Fraisier*   Spanish: *Fresera*)

These leaves make a very invigorating, blood-cleansing drink. They are well suited to take the place of coffee and ordinary tea because they do not irritate the nervous system as do those beverages. They can be used freely and continuously. They aid in alkalinizing the system.

Recent Findings: Fruit extracts of strawberry have been shown to be active against various virus cultures, including influenza, polio, and herpes. The leaf tincture reduced elevated blood sugar in the rat, and a preparation of the entire plant of a related species, *F. virginiana*, demonstrated anti-inflammatory activity in the rat.

Dose: 30–60 grains.

SWEET FLAG
Acorus calamus; part used: the root
(German: *Kalmus*   French: *Acore Odorant*   Spanish: *Calamo Aromatico*)

This well-known stomachic strengthens the digestive organs, increases the appetite, aids the digestion, and prevents the formation of gas and acid in stomach and bowels. Its mild and sure action makes it one of the best-liked stomach remedies. Externally, it is used for applications to boils, indolent ulcers, and open sores.

Recent Findings: Animal and human experiments have amply demonstrated the stimulant properties of sweet flag and its ability to expel gas from the gastrointestinal tract; however, highly concentrated doses might produce undesirable effects. The Food and Drug Administration has banned the use of all varieties of *A. calamus* for human use, on the basis of studies showing that the essential oil induced cancerous growths in rodents to whom it was fed. Only an

Indian variety of the plant was tested in these experiments, and it is known that varieties from other parts of the world differ in their chemical composition from the variety found in India. Nevertheless, a ban is justified until it has been shown that varieties other than the one from India do not have this carcinogenic effect.

Dose: Not recommended. See Recent Findings. Average dose was formerly 15–30 grains.

TORMENTIL
Potentilla erecta; part used: the root
(German: *Tormentil* French: *Tormentille* Spanish: *Tormentilla*)
The powerful astringent properties of this root make it a very valuable remedy in diarrhea, dysentery, internal hemorrhages, etc. The decoction may be used with good results as a douche in leukorrhea (whitish vaginal discharge) and in catarrhal inflammation of the vaginal mucosa, as well as a mouthwash and gargle in inflammation.

Dose: Internally, 30–60 grains.

UVA URSI
Arctostaphylos uva-ursi; part used: the leaves
(German: *Bärentraubenblätter* French: *Bousserole* Spanish: *Gayuba*)
These leaves possess very valuable properties in the treatment of complaints of the urinary tract. The remedy is reputed to be efficacious in dissolving stones in kidneys and bladder and in eliminating uric acid from the blood. It is used in rheumatism and other diseases marked by an accumulation of acids and waste products in the system. It is also used extensively in catarrhal inflammations of the mucous membranes, acute kidney disease, and vaginal discharge.

Recent Findings: Uva Ursi leaves contain *hydroquinone* and *arbutin*, which account for the plant's diuretic, astringent, and urinary antiseptic value. The leaves also contain *allantoin*, which is known to soothe and accelerate the healing of irritated tissues.

Dose: 20–60 grains.

VALERIAN
Valeriana officinalis; part used: the root
(German: *Baldrian*   French: *Racine de Valériane*   Spanish:
Valeriana)

This is a very valuable remedy for nervous disorders. It is extensively used in stomach troubles, palpitations of the heart, sleeplessness, hysteria, headaches, nervous irritability, and other disturbances due to nervousness.

Recent Findings: Recent experiments in Bulgaria showed that an extract of valerian root acted as a sedative on the central nervous system and stabilized irregular heart rhythm in laboratory animals. Experiments in Italy demonstrated that a mixture containing valerian, passionflower, chamomile, and hawthorn was effective in treating children with psychomotor agitation and behavioral disorders.

Dose: 10–15 grains.

VERVAIN
Verbena hastata; part used: the herb
(German: *Eisenkraut*   French: *Verveine*   Spanish: *Verbena*)

This is a very useful remedy in colds and coughs. The hot infusion produces sweating and reduces fever. In complaints of the liver and in indigestion it can be used with good results, and in suppressed menstruation and convulsive disorders, it has been said to have no equal. The infusion used externally in the form of compresses is said to be an effective antidote for poisoning from poison oak and poison ivy. It is one of the most useful simple plants of the herbal kingdom.

Recent Findings: Test-tube studies in China showed the extract of a *Verbena* species to exert a stimulant effect on uterine tissue.

Dose: 15–30 grains.

VIOLET
Viola odorata; part used: the leaves
(German: *Veilchen*   French: *Vilette*   Spanish: *Violeta*)

This well-known tiny plant is valued greatly for its blood-cleansing properties, and in this respect it is hardly surpassed by any other plant. Even if the pollution of the blood has gone quite far, the cleansing effect of its leaves can be noticed quite plainly by its action of loosening mucous obstruction in the inner organs, by its aid in the creation of better blood, and by its aid in improving the resistance of the body.

Dose: 30–60 grains.

WAHOO

Euonymus atropurpurea; part used: the bark of the root
(German: *Spindelbaumrinde*   French: *Écorce d'Evonymus*)

This is a great native American remedy. It stimulates the action of stomach, liver, and bowels. It causes a better flow of the bile and regulates the bowels in a mild but effective way, causing copious stools without pain. In larger doses it is claimed to be very effective in dropsical (fluid retention) conditions.

Dose: 5–8 grains.

WATER CRESS

Nasturtium officinale; part used: the herb
(German: *Brunnenkresse*   French: *Cresson de fontaine*   Spanish: *Berro*)

This plant is rich in iron and other valuable mineral elements. Its blood-purifying and system-cleansing properties cause it to be used extensively as a blood purifier. The green herb is eaten as a salad, while in the dried form it is prepared as a tea.

Recent Findings: Water cress leaf juice was found active against cultures of tubercle bacillus, while Brazilian workers found the plant extract to possess anti-tumor properties when used to treat mice.

Dose: 60 grains.

WATER PEPPER

Polygonum punctatum; part used: the herb
(German: *Americanische Natterwurz*   Spanish: *Chilillo*)

This remedy is reputed to be efficacious in disorders of the urinary organs. It is highly recommended for the removal of stones and gravel in the bladder, as well as for treating suppression of urine and irritation, all caused by increased uric acid.

Recent Findings: For experimental findings for related *Polygonum* species, see the discussion under KNOTGRASS.

Dose: 15 grains.

WHORTLEBERRY

Vaccinium myrtillus; part used: the leaves and berries

(German: *Heidelbeeren*   French: *Myrtille*   Spanish: *Arándano*)

The berries are an excellent remedy in diarrhea, and their juice mixed with water affords a very refreshing drink in all feverish conditions. The leaves are considered one of the best and most reliable remedies in diabetes and also in disorders of the urinary organs, in gravel and stones of the kidneys and bladder.

Recent Findings: Whortleberry plant extracts have been shown in animal studies to have anti-inflammatory activity in the rat, to lower blood sugar in the mouse and the rabbit, and to have capillary anti-hemorrhagic properties in the rabbit. The fruit extract of a related species has shown activity against virus cultures, and in test-tube studies a *Vaccinium* species extract exhibited the ability to coagulate human semen, which suggests a possible contraceptive application.

Dose: Of the leaves, 60 grains several times a day. They should be taken, however, for a long period of time to exert their effect.

WOODRUFF

Asperula odorata; part used: the herb

(German: *Waldemeister*   French: *Asperule*   Spanish: *Enebro*)

This tasty, aromatic little plant is used extensively in Europe in the springtime to make refreshing drinks that stimulate the action of the digestive organs and improve the quality of the blood. Wine or cider is generally used for the extraction, and fresh fruits such as oranges or berries are often added.

Dose: 60 grains.

WORMWOOD

Artemisia absinthium; part used: the herb

(German: *Wermuth*   French: *Absinthe*   Spanish: *Ajenjo*)

Whenever the digestive organs are in a debilitated condition and the liver is sluggish, this herb has no equal in its prompt and reliable action. It promotes the flow of bile in jaundice and other liver complaints. In fever and diarrhea, it also gives excellent results. Its reliable action in expelling worms of stomach and bowels gave the herb its name; since its action is powerful, however, it should be correctly dosed. Externally, it is used as a poultice for swellings, inflammation, bruises, and sprains.

Recent Findings: The essential oil prepared by distilling the herbaceous portions of wormwood is known as absinthe; it is toxic owing to a high concentration of *thujone,* which is a convulsant poison and narcotic in large doses. The use of absinthe is banned in most countries. As an herbal tea, however, wormwood would contain too low a concentration of thujone to be harmful. Although there is no experimental evidence to account for the use of wormwood in expelling intestinal worms, water extracts have been shown to produce a cathartic action in animals. It may be that the bitter properties of wormwood account for its tonic effects through increasing gastric secretion. There is apparently no experimental evidence to support the use of wormwood for bruises, swellings, and inflammations.

Dose: 15–20 grains.

YARROW

Achillea millefolium; part used: the herb
(German: *Schafgarbe*   French: *Milfoil*   Spanish: *Milefolio*)

This is a very useful remedy in menstrual irregularities and hemorrhoids. In catarrhal conditions of the stomach and sluggishness of the liver, it can be used with good results. Its quieting and soothing effect in nervous conditions of the heart also deserve mentioning.

Recent Findings: Decoctions and infusions of yarrow flowers have been given experimentally to humans, and have been shown to stimulate the gastric juices. This would account for yarrow's effectiveness as a tonic, with improved digestion of foods, which is due to the presence of bitter substances in the blossoms. Animal studies have shown that yarrow extracts can reduce inflammation and have a calming effect, and test-tube studies have shown yarrow extracts to have antibiotic properties.

Dose: 30–60 grains.

YELLOW DOCK

Rumex crispus; part used: the root

(German: *Ampferkraut*   French: *Rumex*)

The blood-cleansing properties of this root make it an outstanding remedy in all diseases associated with impurities in the blood. It is therefore especially valuable in skin eruptions, eczema, pimples, boils, rheumatic conditions, and lymph gland enlargement. Its richness in organic iron also improves and enriches the quality of the blood.

Recent Findings: The roots contain a mixture of *anthraquinones* and *anthraquinone glycosides,* similar to those found in cascara sagrada and buckthorn barks; it is these compounds that account for the laxative effect of the roots of yellow dock. The roots also contain *tannins,* which are responsible for the astringent effect of yellow dock preparations applied externally for various skin conditions.

Dose: 60 grains.

YELLOW LADIES' SLIPPER

Cypripedium pubescens; part used: the root

(German: *Frauenschuh Wurzel*   French: *Cypripede jaune*)

The good results obtained from this root in nervous disorders gave it the alternate common name "nerve root." It is used in nervous headaches, nervous irritability, hysteria, spasms, and other disturbances of the nervous system.

Recent Findings: Test-tube studies have demonstrated that the fluidextract was weakly active as a uterine relaxant.

Dose: 15 grains.

7

Materia Medica (Continued):

Other Herbs of Medicinal Value

PLANT NAME		PART	ACTIONS AND	
COMMON	LATIN	USED	USES[*]	DOSAGE[**]
Absinthe—See Wormwood				
Acacia—See Gum Arabic				
Aconite ·	*Aconitum napellus*	Root	Sedative, Anodyne, Poison	1 grain
		Leaves	Sedative, Anodyne, Poison	1 grain
Acorns	*Quercus* spp.	Fruit of Oak	Astringent, Tonic	60 grains

*For definitions of terms in "Actions and Uses" column, see pp. 178–182.
**For equivalent measures, see table of weights and measures, p. 81.

| PLANT NAME | | PART | ACTIONS AND | |
COMMON	LATIN	USED	USES*	DOSAGE**
Agar	*Gracilaria lichenoides*	Plant	Demulcent, Laxative	60 grains
Agaric, White—See Larch Agaric				
Agrimony	*Agrimonia eupatoria*	Herb	Alterative, Stomachic	30–60 grains
Ague Bark—See Wafer Ash				
Ague Root—See Unicorn Root, True				
Ague Weed—See Boneset				
Alder, American—See Tag Alder				
Alder, Black	*Alnus glutinosa*	Bark	Astringent, Tonic	30–60 grains
Alder, Spotted—See Witch Hazel				
Alder, Swamp—See Tag Alder				
Alehoof—See Ground Ivy				
Aletris Root—See Unicorn Root, True				
Alfalfa	*Medicago sativa*	Plant	Rich in vitamins	60 grains
Alkanet	*Alkanna tinctoria*	Root	Colors oils and fats	
All Heal—See Valerian				
Allspice—See Pimento				
Almonds, Bitter	*Amygdalus amara*	Kernels	Sedative	
Almonds, Sweet	*Amygdalus dulcis*	Kernels	Used as food; contains no starch	
		Meal	Used in cosmetics	
Aloe	*Aloe vera* & var. spp.	Gum	Cathartic, Emmenagogue	3–5 grains

*For definitions of terms in "Actions and Uses" column, see pp. 178–182.
**For equivalent measures, see table of weights and measures, p. 81.

PLANT NAME COMMON	LATIN	PART USED	ACTIONS AND USES*	DOSAGE**
		Root	Tonic, Stomachic	15–30 grains
Althaea—See **Marsh Mallow**				
Althaea Rose—See **Hollyhock**				
Alum Root	Heuchera americana	Root	Astringent, Tonic, Vulnerary	15–30 grains
Amadou—See **Larch Agaric**				
Amaranth	Amarantus hypochondriacus	Leaves	Astringent, Detergent	15–30 grains
Ambrette	Abelmoschus moschatus	Seeds	Stomachic, Nervine	5 grains
American Valerian—See **Yellow Ladies' Slipper**				
American Centaury	Sabatia angularis	Plant	Stomachic, Febrifuge, Tonic	30–60 grains
Ammoniac Gum	Dorema ammoniacum	Gum	Expectorant, Counterirritant	5–20 grains
Amoli—See **Soap Bark**				
Anemone, Meadow—See **Meadow Anemone**				
Angelica	Angelica archangelica	Root	Carminative, Stimulant, Aromatic	30–60 grains
		Seeds	Carminative, Stimulant, Aromatic	30–60 grains
Angostura	Galipea jasminiflora	Bark	Tonic, Cathartic, Febrifuge	30–60 grains

*For definitions of terms in "Actions and Uses" column, see pp. 178–182.
**For equivalent measures, see table of weights and measures, p. 81.

PLANT NAME COMMON	LATIN	PART USED	ACTIONS AND USES*	DOSAGE**
Anise	*Pimpinella anisum*	Seed	Carminative, Stimulant, Aromatic	30 grains
Anise, Star—See Star Anise				
Arabic Gum—See Gum Arabic				
Arbor Vitae	*Thuja occidentalis*	Leaves	Stimulant, Diuretic, Emmenagogue	10–15 grains
Archangel—See Angelica				
Areca Nut	*Areca catechu*	Nut	Vermifuge, Astringent	60–120 grains
Arnica	*Arnica montana*	Flowers	Vulnerary, Counterirritant, Diuretic, Stimulant	1–2 grains
		Root	Vulnerary, Counterirritant	5 grains
Arrow, Indian—See Wahoo				
Arrowroot	*Maranta arundinacea*	Root	Nutrient; yields starch	
Asafetida	*Ferula assa-foetida*	Gum	Nervine, Antispasmodic, Stomachic	5–10 grains
Asarabacca	*Asarum europaeum*	Root	Stimulant, Carminative, Diaphoretic	30 grains
Ash, White	*Fraxinus americana*	Bark	Cathartic, Tonic	60 grains
Ash, Black	*Fraxinus nigra*	Bark	Astringent, Tonic	60 grains

*For definitions of terms in "Actions and Uses" column, see pp. 178–182.
**For equivalent measures, see table of weights and measures, p. 81.

PLANT NAME COMMON	LATIN	PART USED	ACTIONS AND USES*	DOSAGE**
Ash, Bitter—See **Quassia**				
Ash, Prickly—See **Prickly Ash**				
Asparagus	*Asparagus officinalis*	Root	Diuretic	60 grains
		Seeds	Diuretic, Aromatic	30–60 grains
Asthma Weed—See **Lobelia**				
Avens Root—See **Water Avens**				
Backache Root—See **Button Snakeroot**				
Balm of Gilead	*Populus balsamifera*	Buds	Vulnerary, Diuretic, Stimulant	60 grains
Balm, Indian—See **Beth Root**				
Balm, Lemon—See **Lemon Balm**				
Balmony	*Chelone glabra*	Herb	Cathartic, Tonic, Anthelmintic	30–60 grains
Balsam Copaiba—See **Copaiba Balsam**				
Balsam Fir	*Abies balsamea*	Bark	Vulnerary, Diuretic	5–10 minims
Balsam, Peru	*Myroxylon balsamum* var. *pereirae*	Balsam	Pectoral, Vulnerary	5–10 minims
Balsam, Tolu	*Myroxylon balsamum*	Balsam	Pectoral, Vulnerary	5–10 minims
Bamboo Brier	*Smilax sarsaparilla*	Root	Alterative, Depurative	30–60 grains
Barberry	*Berberis vulgaris*	Bark of Root	Laxative, Hepatic, Tonic	30 grains
Bardane—See **Burdock**				

*For definitions of terms in "Actions and Uses" column, see pp. 178–182.
**For equivalent measures, see table of weights and measures, p. 81.

237

PLANT NAME COMMON	LATIN	PART USED	ACTIONS AND USES*	DOSAGE**
Basil, Sweet	*Ocimum basilicum*	Herb	Aromatic, Stimulant, Nervine, Spice	30–60 grains
Basket Willow—See Osier Willow				
Basswood	*Tilia americana*	Flowers, Leaves	Antispasmodic, Anodyne	60 grains
Bayberry	*Myrica cerifera*	Bark	Astringent, Stimulant	8–10 grains
Bay Tree	*Laurus nobilis*	Berries	Aromatic, Stomachic, Stimulant	30 grains
		Leaves	Aromatic, Stimulant, Stomachic	30–60 grains
Bearberry Leaves—See Uva Ursi				
Bearberry Bark—See Cascara Sagrada				
Bear's Foot	*Helleborus foetidus*	Leaves	Vermifuge, Emetic	3–5 grains
		Root	Emmenagogue, Purgative	2–3 grains
Bear's Paw—See Male Fern				
Bed Straw—See Cleavers				
Beech Drops	*Orobanche virginiana*	Root	Astringent, Vulnerary	10–30 grains
Beech, European	*Fagus sylvatica*	Leaves	Astringent, Tonic	60–120 grains
Belladonna	*Atropa belladonna*	Leaves	Sedative, Narcotic, Anodyne	1 grain

*For definitions of terms in "Actions and Uses" column, see pp. 178–182.
**For equivalent measures, see table of weights and measures, p. 81.

PLANT NAME COMMON	LATIN	PART USED	ACTIONS AND USES*	DOSAGE**
		Root	Sedative, Narcotic, Anodyne	¾ grain
Benjamin Bush—See **Spicewood**				
Benne—See **Sesame**				
Benzoin, Gum	*Styrax benzoin*	Gum	Pectoral, Antiseptic	15 grains
Betel—See **Areca Nut**				
Beth Root	*Trillium erectum*	Root	Female Complaints, Alterative, Aphrodisiac, Stimulant, Astringent, Tonic, Emmenagogue	30 grains
Betony—See **Wood Betony**				
Bilberry, Black—See **Whortleberry**				
Birch, Black	*Betula lenta*	Bark	Astringent, Stimulant, Diaphoretic, Diuretic	30–60 grains
Bird's Nest Root—See **Wild Carrot**				
Bird Pepper—See **Cayenne Pepper**				
Birth Root—See **Beth Root**				
Bitter Apple—See **Colocynth**				
Bitter Ash Wood—See **Quassia**				
Bitter Bloom—See **Centaury**				
Bitter Orange—See **Orange, Bitter**				

*For definitions of terms in "Actions and Uses" column, see pp. 178–182.
**For equivalent measures, see table of weights and measures, p. 81.

PLANT NAME COMMON	LATIN	PART USED	ACTIONS AND USES*	DOSAGE**
Bitter Root	*Apocynum andro- saemifolium*	Root	Laxative, Diaphoretic, Tonic	5–15 grains
Bittersweet	*Solanum dulcamara*	Root, Twigs	Diuretic, Alterative, Narcotic, Nervine	30–60 grains

Bitter Thistle—See Blessed Thistle
Bitter Wood—See Quassia
Bitterwort Root—See Gentian
Black Alder—See Alder, Black

Blackberry	*Rubus villosus*	Bark of root	Tonic, Astringent (in diarrhea)	15–30 grains

Black Caraway—See Nutmeg Flower

Black Cohosh	*Cimicifuga racemosa*	Root	Nervine, Anti-rheumatic, Diuretic, Tonic	5–30 grains

Black Currant—See Currant, Black
Black Dogwood—See Buckthorn

Black Haw	*Viburnum prunifolium*	Bark of root	Diuretic, Tonic, Antispasmodic, Nervine	30–60 grains

Black Henbane—See Henbane, Black

Black Indian Hemp	*Apocynum cannabinum*	Root	Diaphoretic, Alterative, Cardiac Stimulant	5–15 grains

Black Mustard—See Mustard, Black

*For definitions of terms in "Actions and Uses" column, see pp. 178–182.
**For equivalent measures, see table of weights and measures, p. 81.

PLANT NAME COMMON	LATIN	PART USED	ACTIONS AND USES*	DOSAGE**
Black Root—See **Culver's Root**				
Black Snakeroot—See **Black Cohosh**				
Black Thorn—See **Sloe Tree**				
Bladder Wrack—See **Sea Wrack**				
Blazing Star—See **Button Snakeroot**				
Blessed Thistle	*Cnicus benedictus*	Herb	Stomachic, Febrifuge, Tonic	30–60 grains
Blind Nettle	*Lamium album*	Flowers	Depurative, Styptic	30–60 grains
		Herb	Female complaints, Styptic	60 grains
Blood Root	*Sanguinaria canadensis*	Root	Alterative, Expectorant, Emetic, Sedative, Diuretic	2 grains (Emetic, 15 grains)
Blood Staunch—See **Canada Fleabane**				
Blue Centaury—See **Centaury, Blue**				
Blue Cohosh	*Caulophyllum thalictroides*	Root	Emmenagogue, Antispasmodic, Diuretic	10–30 grains
Blue Flag	*Iris versicolor*	Root	Alterative, Diuretic, Cathartic	15–30 grains
Blue Vervain—See **Vervain**				
Bogbean—See **Buckbean**				
Bog Onion—See **Indian Turnip**				

*For definitions of terms in "Actions and Uses" column, see pp. 178–182.
**For equivalent measures, see table of weights and measures, p. 81.

PLANT NAME COMMON	LATIN	PART USED	ACTIONS AND USES*	DOSAGE**
Boldo	*Peumus boldus*	Leaves	Tonic, Stomachic, Stimulant, Hepatic	5–10 grains
Boneset	*Eupatorium perfoliatum*	Herb	Febrifuge, Diaphoretic, Tonic, Emmenagogue	30–60 grains
Borage	*Borago officinalis*	Flowers	Pectoral, Aperient	60 grains
Boxwood—See **Dogwood, American**				
Bramble	*Rubus fruticosus*	Bark	Astringent (in diarrhea)	15–30 grains
		Leaves	Astringent	60 grains
Brazil Tea—See **Maté**				
Brier Hip—See **Dog Rose**				
Broom	*Cytisus scoparius*	Herb	Diuretic, Cathartic	10–15 grains
Broom Pine	*Pinus palustris*	Oil	Diuretic, Counterirritant	5–10 drops
Bryony, White—See **White Bryony**				
Buchu	*Agathosma crenulata*	Leaves	Diuretic, Tonic	30–60 grains
Buckbean	*Menyanthes trifoliata*	Leaves	Stomachic, Tonic, Febrifuge	20–60 grains
Buckeye—See **Horsechestnut**				

*For definitions of terms in "Actions and Uses" column, see pp. 178–182.
**For equivalent measures, see table of weights and measures, p. 81.

PLANT NAME COMMON	LATIN	PART USED	ACTIONS AND USES*	DOSAGE**
Buckthorn	*Rhamnus cathartica*	Bark	Hepatic, Cathartic	15–30 grains
	Rhamnus frangula	Bark	Hepatic, Cathartic	15–30 grains
		Berries	Cathartic	15–30 grains
Bugleweed	*Lycopus virginicus*	Plant	Astringent, Tonic	30–60 grains
Bugloss Flowers	*Echium vulgare*	Flowers	Aperient, Pectoral	60 grains
Bugloss Root—See **Alkanet**				
Bullsfoot—See **Coltsfoot**				
Burdock	*Arctium lappa*	Root	Diuretic, Alterative, Depurative	60–120 grains
		Seeds	Diuretic, Alterative	30–60 grains
Burgundy Pitch	*Picea excelsa*	Gum	Used in plasters and ointments	
Burning Bush	*Euonymus atropurpurea*	Bark	Laxative, Alterative, Diuretic	8 grains
Butter Bur—See **Coltsfoot**				
Butterfly Weed—See **Pleurisy Root**				
Butternut	*Juglans cinerea*	Bark	Cholagogue, Cathartic, Alterative	30–60 grains

*For definitions of terms in "Actions and Uses" column, see pp. 178–182.
**For equivalent measures, see table of weights and measures, p. 81.

PLANT NAME COMMON	LATIN	PART USED	ACTIONS AND USES*	DOSAGE**
Button Snakeroot	*Liatris spicata*	Root	Tonic, Diuretic, Emmenagogue, Female complaints, Female regulator, Stimulant	15–30 grains
Cacao	*Theobroma cacao*	Beans	A concentrated food; source of cocoa butter, used in ointments and salves	
		Shells	Source of mineral elements	30–60 grains
Cajeput Oil	*Melaleuca leucadendron*	Oil	Carminative, Counterirritant; mostly used in liniments	3–10 drops

Calamus—See **Sweet Flag**
Calendula—See **Marigold**
California Gum Plant—See **Grindelia**
California Poppy—See **Poppy, California**
Calisaya Bark—See **Cinchona, Yellow**
Calumba Root—See **Colombo**

*For definitions of terms in "Actions and Uses" column, see pp. 178–182.
**For equivalent measures, see table of weights and measures, p. 81.

PLANT NAME COMMON	LATIN	PART USED	ACTIONS AND USES*	DOSAGE**
Camphor Tree	*Cinnamonum camphora*	Gum	Sedative, Antiseptic, Rubefacient, Expectorant. Chiefly used in liniments and salves	
Canada Fleabane	*Conyza canadensis*	Herb	Tonic, Astringent, Diuretic	10–30 grains

Canada Snakeroot—See **Snakeroot, Canada**
Cancer Drops—See **Beech Drops**
Cancer Jalap—See **Poke**
Cancer Root—See **Beech Drops**

Canella	*Canella winterana*	Bark	Tonic, Stimulant	10–40 grains

Canker Root—See **Goldthread**
Capsicum—See **Cayenne Pepper**

Caraway	*Carum carvi*	Seeds	Carminative, Aromatic, Spice	30–60 grains
Cardamom	*Elettaria cardamomum*	Seeds	Aromatic, Carminative, Spice	15–30 grains
Carline Thistle	*Carlina acaulis*	Root	Tonic, Emmenagogue	30–60 grains

Carpenter's Square—See **Figwort**
Carrageen—See **Irish Moss**

---

*For definitions of terms in "Actions and Uses" column, see pp. 178–182.
**For equivalent measures, see table of weights and measures, p. 81.

PLANT NAME COMMON	LATIN	PART USED	ACTIONS AND USES*	DOSAGE**
Cascara Sagrada	*Rhamnus purshiana*	Bark	Tonic, Hepatic, Laxative	15–30 grains
Cascarilla	*Croton eluteria*	Bark	Stomachic, Stimulant, Tonic	20–30 grains
Cassia	*Cinnamonum cassia*	Buds	Carminative, Spice	10–20 grains
Cassia Fistula—See Purging Cassia				
Cassia, Purging—See Purging Cassia				
Castor Beans	*Ricinus communis*	Seeds	Poisonous; source of castor oil	
Catarrh Root—See Galanga				
Catechu	*Acacia catechu*	Gum	Astringent, Styptic, Tonic	10 grains
Cat Mint—See Catnip				
Catnip	*Nepeta cataria*	Herb	Antispasmodic, Carminative, Diuretic	30–60 grains
Cat's Foot—See Ground Ivy				
Cayenne Pepper	*Capsicum frutescens*	Fruit	Stimulant, Spice	1–5 grains
Cedar	*Juniperus virginiana*	Wood	Moth destroyer	
Celandine, Great—See Great Celandine				
Celery	*Apium graveolens*	Seeds	Diuretic, Carminative, Spice	20–60 grains
Centaury	*Chironia centaurium*	Herb	Stomachic, Febrifuge, Tonic	30–60 grains

*For definitions of terms in "Actions and Uses" column, see pp. 178–182.
**For equivalent measures, see table of weights and measures, p. 81.

PLANT NAME COMMON	LATIN	PART USED	ACTIONS AND USES*	DOSAGE**
Centaury, American—See American Centaury				
Centaury, Blue	Centaurea cyanus	Flowers	Ophthalmicum, Tonic	30 grains
Ceylon Cinnamon—See Cinnamon, Ceylon				
Chamomile, German	Matricaria chamomilla	Flowers	Carminative, Stomachic, Stimulant	30–60 grains
Chamomile, Roman	Anthemis nobilis	Flowers	Carminative, Stomachic, Stimulant	30–60 grains
Charcoal, Willow	Salix spp.	(Powdered)	Stomachic, Carminative, Absorbent	10–15 grains
Chaulmoogra	Hydnocarpus kurzii	Oil from seed	Used in leprosy	5–10 drops
Cheese Plant—See Low Mallow				
Cherry, Wild	Prunus serotina	Bark	Febrifuge, Sedative (coughs and bronchitis)	30 grains
Chervil	Anthriscus cerefolium	Herb	Esculent, Diuretic, Spice	30–60 grains
Chestnut, American	Castanea dentata	Leaves	Astringent, Pectoral	60 grains
Chia	Salvia chia	Seeds	Mucilaginous	15–30 grains
Chickweed	Stellaria media	Plant	Alterative, Demulcent	30–60 grains
Chickweed, Red—See Red Chickweed				

*For definitions of terms in "Actions and Uses" column, see pp. 178–182.
**For equivalent measures, see table of weights and measures, p. 81.

PLANT NAME COMMON	LATIN	PART USED	ACTIONS AND USES*	DOSAGE**
Chicory	*Cichorium intybus*	Herb	Diuretic, Laxative	60 grains
		Root	Deobstruent, Aperient	60–120 grains
Chili Pepper—See Cayenne Pepper				
China Rhubarb—See Rhubarb				
Chirata	*Swertia chirata*	Herb	Stomachic, Tonic, Hepatic	10–20 grains
Chittam Bark—See Cascara Sagrada				
Chocolate Root—See Water Avens				
Cinchona, Red	*Cinchona pubescens*	Bark	Stomachic, Febrifuge, Tonic	10–60 grains
Cinchona, Yellow	*Cinchona calisaya*	Bark	Stomachic, Febrifuge, Tonic	10–60 grains
Cinnamon, Ceylon	*Cinnamonum verum*	Bark	Stimulant, Carminative, Stomachic, Spice	10–20 grains
Cinnamon, Chinese—See Cassia				
Cleavers	*Galium aparine*	Herb	Aperient, Diuretic	30–60 grains
Clotbur—See Burdock				
Clotweed	*Xanthium spinosum*	Herb	Styptic	30–60 grains
Clove Pepper—See Pimento				
Clover, Crimson	*Trifolium incarnatum*	Flowers	Depurative, Detergent	30–60 grains
Clover, Red	*Trifolium pratense*	Flowers	Depurative, Pectoral	30–60 grains

*For definitions of terms in "Actions and Uses" column, see pp. 178–182.
**For equivalent measures, see table of weights and measures, p. 81.

PLANT NAME COMMON	LATIN	PART USED	ACTIONS AND USES*	DOSAGE**
Clover, White	*Trifolium repens*	Flowers	Depurative, Detergent	30–60 grains
Cloves	*Syzygium aromaticum*	Buds	Stimulant, Spice	5–10 grains
Club Moss	*Lycopodium clavatum*	Spores	Vulnerary (used as dusting powder)	
Coakum Root—See Poke				
Cocillana	*Guarea rusbyi*	Bark	Stomachic, Expectorant	8–15 grains
Cocoa—See Cacao				
Cohosh, Black—See Black Cohosh				
Cohosh, Blue—See Blue Cohosh				
Cola Nut	*Cola acuminata*	Nut	Nervine, Stimulant, Tonic	30–60 grains
Colchicum	*Colchicum autumnale*	Root	Anti-rheumatic, Sedative, Cathartic, Narcotic	2–8 grains
		Seed	Anti-rheumatic, Sedative, Cathartic, Narcotic	2–8 grains
Colic Root—See Button Snakeroot				
Collinsonia	*Collinsonia canadensis*	Root	Stomachic, Diuretic, Vulnerary	15–30 grains
Colocynth Apple	*Citrullus colocynthis*	Fruit pulp	Drastic cathartic	1–5 grains

*For definitions of terms in "Actions and Uses" column, see pp. 178–182.
**For equivalent measures, see table of weights and measures, p. 81.

PLANT NAME COMMON	LATIN	PART USED	ACTIONS AND USES*	DOSAGE**
Colombo	Jateorhiza palmata	Root	Stomachic, Tonic	10–30 grains
Coltsfoot	Tussilago farfara	Leaves	Expectorant, Demulcent, Tonic	60–120 grains
Comfrey	Symphytum officinale	Root	Pectoral, Demulcent, Tonic	30–60 grains

Cone Flower, Purple—See Echinacea
Consumptive Weed—See Yerba Santa
Convulsion Weed—See Ice Plant

Coolwort	Tiarella cordifolia	Leaves	Diuretic	10–30 grains
Copaiba Balsam	Copaifera officinalis	Oleo-resin	Diuretic, Astringent, Expectorant	5–15 minims
Copal Gum	Agathis oranthifolia	Gum	Used in varnishes	
Copalchi	Croton pseudo-china	Bark	Febrifuge, Stomachic	10–60 grains
Coriander	Coriandrum sativum	Seeds	Stimulant, Carminative, Spice	20–60 grains
Corn	Zea mays	Silk	Diuretic, Lithotropic	60–120 grains
Cotton	Gossypium herbaceum	Bark of root	Emmenagogue, Diuretic	30–60 grains
Couch Grass	Agropyron repens	Root	Diuretic, Nephritic, Depurative	60–120 grains

Coughwort—See Coltsfoot

---

*For definitions of terms in "Actions and Uses" column, see pp. 178–182.
**For equivalent measures, see table of weights and measures, p. 81.

PLANT NAME COMMON	LATIN	PART USED	ACTIONS AND USES*	DOSAGE**
Cowslip	*Primula veris*	Flowers	Antispasmodic, Nervine, Tonic	15–30 grains
Cramp Bark	*Viburnum opulus*	Bark	Anti-periodic, Antispasmodic, Alterative	30–60 grains
Cranberry, Mountain—See Uva Ursi				
Cranesbill	*Geranium maculatum*	Root	Astringent, Tonic, Styptic	20–30 grains
Crawley Root	*Corallorhiza odontorhiza*	Root	Febrifuge, Diaphoretic	15–30 grains
Crow Corn—See Unicorn Root, True				
Cubeb	*Piper cubeba*	Berries	Diuretic, Stimulant	10–60 grains
Cucumber Tree	*Magnolia acuminata*	Bark	Febrifuge, Stimulant	30–60 grains
Cudbear—See Tartarean Moss				
Culver's Root	*Veronica virginica*	Root	Laxative, Cholagogue, Hepatic, Tonic	15–60 grains
Cumin	*Cuminum cyminum*	Seeds	Stimulant, Spice	15–30 grains
Curcuma Root—See Turmeric				
Cure All Root—See Water Avens				
Currant, Black	*Ribes nigrum*	Leaves	Expectorant, Diuretic	30–60 grains
Daisy	*Bellis perennis*	Leaves	Vulnerary, Antiscorbutic	30–60 grains
Dalmatian Insect Powder	*Chrysanthemum cinerariifolium*	Flowers	Insecticide	

*For definitions of terms in "Actions and Uses" column, see pp. 178–182.
**For equivalent measures, see table of weights and measures, p. 81.

PLANT NAME COMMON	LATIN	PART USED	ACTIONS AND USES*	DOSAGE**
Damiana	*Turnera diffusa*	Leaves	Aphrodisiac, Tonic, Stimulant	30–60 grains
Dammar Resin	*Shorea robusta*	Resin	Used in varnishes, plasters	
Dandelion	*Taraxacum officinale*	Leaves	Hepatic, Depurative, Tonic	30–60 grains
		Root	Depurative, Diuretic, Hepatic, Stimulant	60–120 grains
Deadly Nightshade—See **Belladonna**				
Deer Tongue—See **Vanilla Leaf**				
Devil's Apple—See **Stramonium**				
Devil's Bit—See **Button Snakeroot**				
Devil's Shoe Strings—See **Hoary Pea**				
Digitalis—See **Foxglove**				
Dill	*Anethum graveolens*	Seeds	Stimulant, Carminative, Spice	30–60 grains
Dittany	*Cunila origanoides*	Herb	Antispasmodic, Nervine, Stimulant	30–60 grains
Dittany of Crete	*Amaracus dictamnus*	Herb	Tonic, Aromatic	30–60 grains
Dock, Yellow—See **Yellow Dock**				
Dog Grass—See **Couch Grass**				
Dog Rose	*Rosa canina*	Fruit	Diuretic, Antilithic	30–60 grains

*For definitions of terms in "Actions and Uses" column, see pp. 178–182.
**For equivalent measures, see table of weights and measures, p. 81.

PLANT NAME COMMON	LATIN	PART USED	ACTIONS AND USES*	DOSAGE**
		Seeds	Diuretic	30–60 grains
Dogwood, American	*Cornus florida*	Bark	Tonic, Astringent, Emmenagogue	60–120 grains
Dogwood, Jamaica	*Piscidia erythrina*	Bark	Narcotic, Soporific	30–60 grains
Double Tansy—See Tansy				
Doves Foot	*Geranium sylvaticum*	Herb	Astringent, Tonic, Styptic	20–30 grains
Dragon Root—See Indian Turnip				
Dragon's Blood	*Calamus draco*	Extract	Colors red	
Dropsy Plant—See Lemon Balm				
Dulse	*Rhodymenia palmata*	Sea plant	Alterative, Antifat. Contains organic iodine.	10–60 grains
Dwarf Elder	*Sambucus ebulus*	Root	Diaphoretic, Diuretic	15–30 grains
Dwarf Nettle	*Urtica urens*	Plant	Diuretic, Depurative, Stimulant, Pectoral	30–60 grains
Dyer's Broom	*Genista tinctoria*	Tops	Diuretic. Dyes yellow	10–15 grains
Echinacea	*Echinacea pallida*	Root	Alterative, Anti-syphilitic	15–30 grains
Elder	*Sambucus canadensis, S. nigra*	Berries	Diuretic, Aperient	30–60 grains

*For definitions of terms in "Actions and Uses" column, see pp. 178–182.
**For equivalent measures, see table of weights and measures, p. 81.

PLANT NAME COMMON	LATIN	PART USED	ACTIONS AND USES*	DOSAGE**
Elder (continued)		Bark	Purgative	30 grains
		Flowers	Diaphoretic, Depurative	30–60 grains
		Leaves	Diaphoretic, Depurative	60 grains
Elecampane	*Inula helenium*	Root	Expectorant, Diuretic, Stimulant	20–60 grains
Elm, Slippery—See **Slippery Elm**				
Ephedra	*Ephedra trifurca* and var. spp.	Herb	Expectorant	60 grains
Eryngo, Wild	*Eryngium campestre*	Root	Diuretic, Sudorific	15–30 grains
Eschscholtzia—See **Poppy, California**				
Estragon—See **Tarragon**				
Eucalyptus	*Eucalyptus globulus*	Leaves	Febrifuge, Anti-periodic	10–30 grains
Euphorbium	*Euphorbia canariensis*	Herb	Depurative, Cathartic	30 grains
European Buckthorn—See **Buckthorn**				
Evans Root—See **Water Avens**				
Eyebright	*Euphrasia officinalis*	Herb	Astringent, Tonic, Stomachic	60 grains
False Hellebore—See **Hellebore, White**				
False Unicorn Root—See **Helonias**				
Febrifuge Plant—See **Fever Few**				
Felonwort—See **Bittersweet**				
Female Regulator Plant—See **Life Root**				

*For definitions of terms in "Actions and Uses" column, see pp. 178–182.
**For equivalent measures, see table of weights and measures, p. 81.

PLANT NAME COMMON	LATIN	PART USED	ACTIONS AND USES[*]	DOSAGE[**]
Fennel	Foeniculum vulgare	Seeds	Carminative, Stomachic	30–60 grains
Fenugreek	Trigonella foenumgraecum	Seeds	Anti-phlogistic, Mucilaginous for poultices	60 grains
Fever Bush—See **Spicewood**				
Fever Few	Chrysanthemum parthenium	Herb	Febrifuge, Stimulant, Carminative	30–60 grains
Feverwort—See **Boneset**				
Figwort	Scrophularia nodosa	Herb	Alterative, Diuretic, Female complaints	30–60 grains
Fireweed—See **Canada Fleabane**				
Fit Plant—See **Ice Plant**				
Flag, Blue—See **Blue Flag**				
Flag, Sweet—See **Sweet Flag**				
Flax Seed	Linum usitatissimum	Seeds	Emollient, Pectoral, Mucilaginous, Nephritic	60–120 grains
Fleabane, Canada—See **Canada Fleabane**				
Fleaseed—See **Psyllium**				
Foenum Graecum Seed—See **Fenugreek**				
Foxglove	Digitalis purpurea	Leaves	Diuretic, Sedative, Narcotic (in heart diseases)	1–2 grains
Frankincense—See **Olibanum**				

[*]For definitions of terms in "Actions and Uses" column, see pp. 178–182.
[**]For equivalent measures, see table of weights and measures, p. 81.

Materia Medica (continued)

PLANT NAME COMMON	LATIN	PART USED	ACTIONS AND USES*	DOSAGE**
Friar's Cap—See Aconite				
Fringe Tree	Chionanthus virginica	Bark	Diuretic, Tonic, Febrifuge	30–60 grains
Frostwort	Helianthemum canadense	Herb	Tonic, Astringent, Depurative	30–60 grains
Fumitory	Fumaria officinalis	Leaves	Laxative, Diuretic, Alterative	60 grains
Galanga	Alpinia galanga	Root	Stomachic, Stimulant	15–30 grains
Galbanum Gum	Ferula gummosa	Gum	Expectorant, Counterirritant	5–10 grains
Gambir—See Catechu				
Gamboge	Garcinia hanburyi	Gum resin	Drastic Cathartic	1–3 grains
Garden Celandine—See Great Celandine				
Garden Lettuce—See Lettuce, Garden				
Garget Root—See Poke				
Gay Feather Root—See Button Snakeroot				
Gelsemium—See Yellow Jessamine				
Genepi	Artemisia laxa	Herb	Aromatic, Stomachic, Stimulant	30–60 grains
Gentian, Blue	Gentiana catesbaei	Root	Stomachic, Tonic, Anti-bilious, Anthelmintic	15 grains

*For definitions of terms in "Actions and Uses" column, see pp. 178–182.
**For equivalent measures, see table of weights and measures, p. 81.

PLANT NAME COMMON	LATIN	PART USED	ACTIONS AND USES*	DOSAGE**
Gentian, Yellow	*Gentiana lutea*	Root	Stomachic, Tonic	15 grains
Geranium, Spotted—See **Cranesbill**				
German Chamomile—See **Chamomile, German**				
Germander	*Teucrium chamaedrys*	Herb	Hepatic, Stimulant, Febrifuge	30 grains
Gillrun—See **Ground Ivy**				
Ginger	*Zingiber officinale*	Root	Stomachic, Stimulant, Spice	10–20 grains
Ginseng	*Panax quinquefolia* and var. spp.	Root	Stimulant, Tonic	15–30 grains
Goat's Foot—See **Gout Weed**				
Golden Rod, European	*Solidago virgaurea*	Herb	Astringent, Diuretic, Antilithic	60 grains
Golden Seal	*Hydrastis canadensis*	Root	Anodyne, Tonic, Hepatic	15–30 grains
Goldthread	*Coptis trifolia*	Root	Astringent (in canker sores)	10–30 grains
Goose Grass—See **Cleavers**				
Gout Weed	*Aegopodium podagraria*	Root	Anti-rheumatic, Diuretic	30 grains
Grains of Paradise	*Aframomum sceptrum*	Seeds	Aromatic, Stimulant, Pungent Spice	15–30 grains
Grass Myrtle—See **Sweet Flag**				

*For definitions of terms in "Actions and Uses" column, see pp. 178–182.
**For equivalent measures, see table of weights and measures, p. 81.

PLANT NAME COMMON	LATIN	PART USED	ACTIONS AND USES*	DOSAGE**
Gravel Plant—See **Trailing Arbutus**				
Great Celandine	*Chelidonium majus*	Herb	Cathartic, Diuretic, Diaphoretic, Stimulant	15–60 grains
Green Ozier	*Cornus circinnata*	Bark	Astringent, Tonic	60 grains
Grindelia	*Grindelia robusta*	Herb	Antispasmodic, Demulcent	30–40 grains
Ground Holly—See **Pipsissewa**				
Ground Ivy	*Glechoma hederacea*	Herb	Tonic, Pectoral, Stimulant, Diuretic	30–60 grains
Ground Laurel—See **Trailing Arbutus**				
Guaiac	*Guaiacum officinale*	Wood	Alterative, Diuretic, Anti-rheumatic, Stimulant	60 grains
		Gum resin	Alterative, Diuretic, Anti-rheumatic, Stimulant	10–30 grains
Guarana	*Paullinia cupana*	Extract from seeds	Stimulant, Nervine	20–60 grains
Gum Acacia— See **Gum Arabic**				
Gum Aloe—See **Aloe**				
Gum Arabic	*Acacia senegal*	Gum	Mucilaginous, Demulcent	½ ounce
Gum Asafetida—See **Asafetida**				

*For definitions of terms in "Actions and Uses" column, see pp. 178–182.
**For equivalent measures, see table of weights and measures, p. 81.

PLANT NAME		PART	ACTIONS AND	
COMMON	LATIN	USED	USES*	DOSAGE**

Gum Benzoin—See **Benzoin, Gum**

Gum Camphor—See **Camphor Tree**

Gum Catechu—See **Catechu**

Gum Guaiac—See **Guaiac**

Gum Myrrh—See **Myrrh**

Gum Olibanum—See **Olibanum**

Gum Sandarac—See **Sandarac**

Gum Spruce—See **Spruce, Black**

Gum Tragacanth—See **Tragacanth**

Gum Tree	*Liquidambar styraciflua*	Leaves	Febrifuge, Stomachic	10–30 grains

Haw, Black—See **Black Haw**

Hawthorn, English	*Crataegus oxyacantha*	Berries	Astringent	60 grains

Heartsease—See **Pansy**

Hedge Hyssop	*Gratiola officinalis*	Herb	Cathartic, Diuretic, Narcotic	15–30 grains

Hedge Maids' Herb—See **Ground Ivy**

Hellebore, White	*Veratrum viride*	Root	Respiratory and Heart Sedative	1–2 grains
Helonias	*Chamaelirium luteum*	Root	Alterative, Diuretic, Tonic, Vermifuge, Female regulator	15–30 grains
Hemlock Spruce	*Tsuga canadensis*	Bark	Tonic, Astringent	30–60 grains

Hemp—See **Marijuana**

---

*For definitions of terms in "Actions and Uses" column, see pp. 178–182.
**For equivalent measures, see table of weights and measures, p. 81.

PLANT NAME COMMON	LATIN	PART USED	ACTIONS AND USES*	DOSAGE**
Hemp, Black Indian—See **Black Indian Hemp**				
Hemp Nettle	*Galeopsis tetrahit*	Herb	Expectorant	30–60 grains
Henbane, Black	*Hyoscyamus niger*	Herb	Nervine, Narcotic, Anodyne, Antispasmodic	2–5 grains
Henna	*Lawsonia inermis*	Leaves	Colors hair	
Hickory	*Carya laciniosa*	Bark	Astringent	30 grains
Hip Fruit—See **Dog Rose**				
Hip Seed—See **Dog Rose**				
Hoarhound—See **Horehound**				
Hoary Pea	*Tephrosia virginiana*	Root	Anti-syphilitic, Stimulant	30–60 grains
Holly, European	*Ilex aquifolium*	Leaves	Tonic, Stimulant, Astringent	30 grains
Hollyhock	*Althaea rosea*	Flowers	Demulcent, Emmenagogue	30 grains
Holly-Leaved Barberry—See **Oregon Grape Root**				
Holy Thistle—See **Blessed Thistle**				
Honey Bloom Root—See **Bitter Root**				
Honey Bread Fruit—See **Saint John's Bread**				
Hops	*Humulus lupulus*	Flowers	Nervine, Anodyne, Febrifuge	30–90 grains
Horehound	*Marrubium vulgare*	Herb	Expectorant, Tonic	30–60 grains

*For definitions of terms in "Actions and Uses" column, see pp. 178–182.
**For equivalent measures, see table of weights and measures, p. 81.

PLANT NAME COMMON	LATIN	PART USED	ACTIONS AND USES*	DOSAGE**
Horsechestnut	*Aesculus hippocastanum*	Seeds	Astringent, Febrifuge	15–30 grains
		Leaves	Expectorant, Stimulant	60 grains
Horsefly Weed—See **Wild Indigo**				
Horse Heal—See **Elecampane**				
Horse Mint	*Monarda punctata*	Herb	Emmenagogue, Stimulant, Diuretic	30 grains
Horse Nettle	*Solanum carolinense*	Herb	Anodyne, Narcotic	30–60 grains
		Berries	Alterative	30–60 grains
Horse Pipe—See **Scouring Rush**				
Horse Radish	*Armoracia rusticana*	Root	Tonic, Diuretic, Stomachic	5–10 grains
Horse Tail—See **Scouring Rush**				
Huckleberry	*Gaylussacia baccata*	Dried berries	Antiseptic, Astringent (in diarrhea)	60–120 grains
		Leaves	Diuretic (in diabetes)	60 grains
Hydrangea	*Hydrangea arborescens*	Root, Leaves	Antilithic, Diuretic	15–30 grains
Hydrocotyle, Asiatic—See **Indian Pennywort**				
Hyssop	*Hyssopus officinalis*	Herb	Aromatic, Pectoral, Stimulant	60 grains

*For definitions of terms in "Actions and Uses" column, see pp. 178–182.
**For equivalent measures, see table of weights and measures, p. 81.

| PLANT NAME | | PART | ACTIONS AND | |
COMMON	LATIN	USED	USES*	DOSAGE**
Iceland Moss	*Cetraria islandica*	Plant	Expectorant, Demulcent	30–60 grains
Ice Plant	*Monotropa uniflora*	Root	Nervine, Sedative, Antispasmodic	15–30 grains

Indian Apple Root—See **Mandrake**
Indian Arrow Root—See **Wahoo**
Indian Balm Root—See **Beth Root**
Indian Chocolate Root—See **Water Avens**
Indian Elm—See **Slippery Elm**
Indian Ginger Root—See **Snakeroot, Canada**
Indian Hemp, Black—See **Black Indian Hemp**

Indian Pennywort	*Centella asiatica*	Plant	Diuretic, Aromatic, Astringent, Stimulant	10–30 grains
Indian Physic Root	*Gillenia trifoliata*	Root	Diuretic, Cathartic, Emmenagogue	5–15 grains

Indian Pink Root—See **Pink Root**
Indian Root—See **Spikenard**
Indian Sage—See **Boneset**
Indian Tobacco—See **Lobelia**

Indian Turnip	*Arisaema triphyllum*	Root	Diaphoretic, Expectorant, Stimulant	10–30 grains

Indigo Broom—See **Wild Indigo**

Indigo Plant	*Indigofera tinctoria*	Leaves	Dyes blue	

Indigo, Wild—See **Wild Indigo**
Inkroot—See **Marsh Rosemary**

---

*For definitions of terms in "Actions and Uses" column, see pp. 178–182.
**For equivalent measures, see table of weights and measures, p. 81.

PLANT NAME COMMON	LATIN	PART USED	ACTIONS AND USES*	DOSAGE**
Insect Powder, Dalmatian—See **Dalmatian Insect Powder**				
Ipecac	*Cephaelis ipecacuanha*	Root	Emetic	⅙–1 grain
			Expectorant	15–30 grains
Irish Moss	*Chondrus crispus*	Sea plant	Expectorant, Demulcent, Mucilaginous, Nutrient	60–240 grains
Jaborandi	*Piper longum*	Leaves	Diaphoretic	30–60 grains
Jack in the Pulpit—See **Indian Turnip**				
Jalap	*Ipomoea purga*	Root	Hydragogue Cathartic, Diuretic	10–30 grains
Jamaica Dogwood—See **Dogwood, Jamaica**				
Jambul	*Eugenia jambolana*	Seeds	Diuretic, Astringent	60 grains
Jamestown Weed—See **Stramonium**				
Jaundice Root—See **Golden Seal**				
Java Tea	*Orthosiphon stamineus*	Leaves	Diuretic	30–60 grains
Jequirity—See **Love Pea**				
Jersey Tea—See **Red Root**				
Jerusalem Oak	*Chenopodium botrys*	Flowers	Anthelmintic, Antispasmodic	20–60 grains
Jessamine, Yellow—See **Yellow Jessamine**				
Jesuit's Bark—See **Cinchona**				
Jimson Weed—See **Stramonium**				
Job's Tears	*Coix lacryma-jobi*	Seeds	Used as beads; Diuretic, Tonic	

*For definitions of terms in "Actions and Uses" column, see pp. 178–182.
**For equivalent measures, see table of weights and measures. p. 81.

PLANT NAME COMMON	LATIN	PART USED	ACTIONS AND USES*	DOSAGE**
John'swort—See Saint John'swort				
Juniper	*Juniperus communis*	Berries	Diuretic, Carminative	60 grains
		Twigs	Diuretic, Carminative	60 grains
Kameela	*Mallotus philippensis*	Fruit, powdered	Vermifuge	60–180 grains
Karaya Gum	*Sterculia urens*	Gum	Demulcent, Mucilaginous (in hair setting)	
Kava Kava	*Piper methysticum*	Root	Diuretic	15–45 grains
Kelp—See Sea Wrack				
Kidney Liverwort—See Liverwort				
Kidney Root—See Queen of the Meadow				
Kinnikinnick Bark—See Swamp Dogwood				
Kinnikinnick Leaves—See Uva Ursi				
Kino	*Pterocarpus marsupium*	Extract	Astringent	10–30 grains
Knot Grass	*Polygonum aviculare*	Plant	Diuretic, Depurative	60 grains
Kola Nut—See Cola Nut				
Kousso	*Hagenia abyssinica*	Flowers	Anthelmintic for tapeworm	120–240 grains
Ladies' Slipper—See Yellow Ladies' Slipper				
Lady's Mantle	*Alchemilla vulgaris*	Plant	Astringent, Styptic	60 grains
Larch Agaric	*Polyporus officinalis*	Fungus	Cathartic, Astringent, Emetic, Styptic	120–240 grains

*For definitions of terms in "Actions and Uses" column, see pp. 178–182.
**For equivalent measures, see table of weights and measures, p. 81.

PLANT NAME COMMON	LATIN	PART USED	ACTIONS AND USES*	DOSAGE**
Larkspur	*Consolida regalis*	Seeds	Parasiticide, Poison	
Laurel, European—See **Bay Tree**				
Lavender	*Lavandula officinalis*	Flowers	Carminative, Stimulant, Aromatic	10–30 grains
Lemon Balm	*Melissa officinalis*	Herb	Antispasmodic, Carminative, Diaphoretic, Astringent, Tonic, Styptic	60 grains
Leopard's Bane—See **Arnica**				
Leptandra—See **Culver's Root**				
Lettuce, Garden	*Lactuca sativa*	Leaves	Soothing to the nerves	60 grains
Lettuce, Wild	*Lactuca elongata*	Herb	Hypnotic, Narcotic, Diuretic	10–20 grains
Licorice	*Glycyrrhiza glabra*	Root	Expectorant, Demulcent	60–240 grains
Life Everlasting	*Gnaphalium polycephalum*	Herb	Astringent, Diaphoretic	30–60 grains
Life Root	*Senecio aureus*	Herb	Emmenagogue, Female regulator, Diuretic, Diaphoretic	30–60 grains
Lily of the Valley	*Convallaria majalis*	Root	Heart Tonic, Poison	5–10 grains
Lime Tree—See **Basswood**				

*For definitions of terms in "Actions and Uses" column, see pp. 178–182.
**For equivalent measures, see table of weights and measures, p. 81.

| PLANT NAME | | PART | ACTIONS AND | |
COMMON	LATIN	USED	USES*	DOSAGE**
Linden	*Tilia europaea*	Flowers	Antispasmodic, Nervine	60 grains
Linseed—See Flax Seed				
Lion's Tail—See Motherwort				
Lion's Tooth—See Dandelion				
Liver Lily—See Blue Flag				
Liver Weed—See Liverwort				
Liverwort	*Hepatica americana*	Herb	Pectoral, Astringent, Hepatic	30–60 grains
Lobelia	*Lobelia inflata*	Herb	Antispasmodic, Emetic, Expectorant, Diaphoretic	1–5 grains
Locust Bean—See Saint John's Bread				
Logwood	*Haematoxylum campechianum*	Wood	Dyestuff	
		Extract	Astringent, Tonic	
Long Pepper—See Jaborandi				
Lovage	*Levisticum officinale*	Root	Stomachic, Aromatic, Carminative, Diuretic	10–30 grains
Love Pea	*Abrus precatorius*	Seeds	Used as beads	
		Root, Leaves	Pectoral, Mucilaginous, Demulcent	

*For definitions of terms in "Actions and Uses" column, see pp. 178–182.
**For equivalent measures, see table of weights and measures, p. 81.

PLANT NAME COMMON	LATIN	PART USED	ACTIONS AND USES*	DOSAGE**
Low Mallow	*Malva pusilla*	Herb	Emollient, Diuretic, Demulcent	60 grains
Lung Moss	*Sticta pulmonaria*	Plant	Expectorant, Demulcent	30–60 grains
Lungwort	*Pulmonaria officinalis*	Herb	Pectoral, Demulcent	60 grains
Lycopodium—See **Club Moss**				
Mace—See **Nutmeg**				
Madder Root	*Rubia tinctorium*	Root	Deobstruent, Diuretic, Emmenagogue, a dyestuff	60 grains
Mad Dog Weed—See **Water Plantain**				
Mahogany, Mountain—See **Birch, Black**				
Ma-huang	*Ephedra sinica*	Herb	Expectorant, Bronchodilator	60 grains
Maidenhair	*Adiantum pedatum*	Herb	Expectorant, Tonic, Astringent	60 grains
Male Fern	*Aspidium filix mas*	Root	Anthelmintic	60–120 grains
Mallow	*Malva sylvestris*	Flowers	Demulcent, Emollient, Pectoral	60 grains
		Leaves	Demulcent, Diuretic	60 grains
Mallow, Low—See **Low Mallow**				
Malva—See **Mallow**				

*For definitions of terms in "Actions and Uses" column, see pp. 178–182.
**For equivalent measures, see table of weights and measures, p. 81.

PLANT NAME COMMON	LATIN	PART USED	ACTIONS AND USES*	DOSAGE**
Malva, Black—See Hollyhock				
Manaca	*Franciscea uniflora*	Root	Anti-rheumatic, Deobstruent	10–30 grains
Mandrake	*Podophyllum peltatum*	Root	Hepatic, Anthelmintic, Cholagogue, Alterative	5–10 grains
Manna	*Fraxinus ornus*	Exudate	Mild laxative	120–240 grains
Mare's Tail—See Scouring Rush				
Marigold	*Calendula officinalis*	Flowers	Stimulant, Diaphoretic, Vulnerary	15–60 grains
Marijuana	*Cannabis sativa*	Flowering tops	Hypnotic, Antispasmodic, Sedative, Anodyne, Nervine, Stimulant	As needed
Marjoram, Sweet—See Sweet Marjoram				
Marjoram, Wild	*Origanum vulgare*	Herb	Tonic, Aromatic, Stimulant	30–60 grains
Marsh Clover—See Buckbean				
Marsh Mallow	*Althaea officinalis*	Root	Expectorant, Demulcent, Mucilaginous	30–60 grains
		Herb	Expectorant, Demulcent, Mucilaginous	60 grains

*For definitions of terms in "Actions and Uses" column, see pp. 178–182.
**For equivalent measures, see table of weights and measures, p. 81.

Materia Medica (continued)

PLANT NAME COMMON	LATIN	PART USED	ACTIONS AND USES*	DOSAGE**
Marsh Rosemary	Statice limonium	Root	Astringent	30–60 grains
Marsh Tea	Ledum palustre	Leaves	Tonic, Astringent	15–30 grains
Maryland Pink—See Pink Root				
Masterwort, Imperial	Astrantia major, Imperatoria ostruthium	Root	Stimulant, Aromatic	10–15 grains
Mastic	Pistacia lentiscus	Oil	Antispasmodic; Gum used in varnishes	
Maté	Ilex paraguayensis	Leaves	Tonic, Stimulant; Used as tea	60 grains
Matico	Artanthe elongata	Leaves	Stimulant, Vulnerary, Styptic	40–70 grains
May Apple—See Mandrake				
Meadow Anemone	Anemone pulsatilla	Herb	Heart Sedative	2–20 grains
Meadow Saffron—See Colchicum				
Meadow Sweet	Filipendula ulmaria	Leaves	Diuretic	60 grains
Melilot, White	Melilotus alba	Flowers	Emollient, Diuretic	60 grains
Mercury Herb	Mercurialis annua	Herb	Purgative, Discutient	15–30 grains
Mezereon	Daphne mezereum	Bark	Irritant, Diuretic, Narcotic	10 grains

*For definitions of terms in "Actions and Uses" column, see pp. 178–182.
**For equivalent measures, see table of weights and measures, p. 81.

| PLANT NAME | | PART | ACTIONS AND | |
COMMON	LATIN	USED	USES*	DOSAGE**
Milfoil—See **Yarrow**				
Milkweed	*Asclepias syriaca*	Root	Laxative, Tonic, Diuretic	20–60 grains
Millefolium—See **Yarrow**				
Mint—See **Spearmint**				
Mistletoe	*Viscum album*	Herb	Styptic, Antispasmodic, Female regulator	30 grains
Moccasin Plant—See **Yellow Ladies' Slipper**				
Moon Seed—See **Yellow Parilla**				
Motherwort	*Leonorus cardiaca*	Herb	Expectorant, Female regulator	30–60 grains
Mountain Ash, American	*Sorbus americana*	Leaves	Tonic, Astringent	60 grains
Mountain Ash, European	*Sorbus aucuparia*	Leaves	Tonic, Astringent	60 grains
Mountain Balm—See **Yerba Santa**				
Mountain Cranberry—See **Uva Ursi**				
Mountain Dittany—See **Dittany**				
Mountain Mahogany—See **Birch, Black**				
Mountain Pink—See **Trailing Arbutus**				
Mountain Rush	*Ephedra antisyphilitica*	Stem	Stimulant, Antispasmodic, Anti-syphilitic	60 grains
Mountain Sage—See **Sage, Mountain**				
Mouse Bloodwort	*Hieracium pilosella*	Plant	Astringent, Febrifuge	30 grains
Mouse Ear—See **Mouse Bloodwort**				
Mouth Root—See **Goldthread**				

*For definitions of terms in "Actions and Uses" column, see pp. 178–182.
**For equivalent measures, see table of weights and measures, p. 81.

PLANT NAME COMMON	LATIN	PART USED	ACTIONS AND USES*	DOSAGE**
Mugwort	*Artemisia vulgaris*	Herb	Stomachic, Emmenagogue, Nervine, Spice	60 grains
Muirapuama	*Liriosma ovata*	Root	Aphrodisiac, Stimulant	15–30 grains
Mullein	*Verbascum thapsus*	Flowers	Demulcent, Pectoral	60 grains
		Leaves	Demulcent, Antispasmodic, Diuretic	60 grains
Murillo Bark—See **Soap Bark**				
Musk Root	*Euryangium sumbul*	Root	Nervine, Stimulant, Tonic, Stomachic	15–30 grains
Musk Seed—See **Ambrette**				
Mustard, Black	*Brassica nigra*	Seeds	Irritant, Emetic, Anti-rheumatic	60–150 grains
Mustard, White (Yellow)	*Sinapis alba*	Seeds	Stimulant, Spice	
Myrrh	*Commiphora myrrha*	Gum	Astringent, Vulnerary, Expectorant	10–30 grains
Myrtle Flag—See **Sweet Flag**				
Nasturtium—See **Water Cress**				
Nerve Root	*Cypripedium flavum*	Root	Nervine, Antispasmodic	15 grains
Nest Root—See **Ice Plant**				
Nettle, Blind—See **Blind Nettle**				

*For definitions of terms in "Actions and Uses" column, see pp. 178–182.
**For equivalent measures, see table of weights and measures, p. 81.

| PLANT NAME | | PART | ACTIONS AND | |
COMMON	LATIN	USED	USES*	DOSAGE**
Nettle, Dwarf—See **Dwarf Nettle**				
New Jersey Tea—See **Red Root**				
Nigella—See **Nutmeg Flower**				
Night-Blooming Cereus	*Silenicereus grandiflorus*	Flowers	Diuretic, Sedative	5–15 grains
Nightshade—See **Bittersweet**				
Nutgalls	*Quercus infectoria*	Galls	Astringent, Styptic	5–15 grains
Nutmeg	*Myristica fragrans*	Kernels of fruit	Stimulant, Stomachic, Spice	5–20 grains
Nutmeg Flower	*Nigella sativa*	Plant	Expectorant, Sialagogue, Spice	
Oak, Red	*Quercus rubra*	Bark	Astringent, Styptic	15–60 grains
Oak, White	*Quercus alba*	Bark	Astringent, Styptic	15–60 grains
Oats	*Avena sativa*	Straw	Contains silicon	60 grains
Oleander	*Nerium oleander*	Leaves	Herpetic, Vulnerary	1–3 grains
Olibanum	*Boswellia carteri*	Gum	Aromatic; Church incense	
Orange	*Citrus sinensis*	Flowers	Aromatic, Nervine	30–60 grains
		Leaves	Aromatic, Diaphoretic	60 grains

*For definitions of terms in "Actions and Uses" column, see pp. 178–182.
**For equivalent measures, see table of weights and measures, p. 81.

PLANT NAME COMMON	LATIN	PART USED	ACTIONS AND USES*	DOSAGE**
		Peel	Aromatic, Stomachic	30–60 grains
Orange, Bitter	*Citrus aurantium*	Peel	Stomachic, Tonic (in cordials)	15–60 grains
Oregon Grape Root	*Mahonia aquifolium*	Root	Hepatic, Tonic, Anti-rheumatic	30–60 grains
Orris Root	*Iris florentina*	Root	Cathartic, Febrifuge, Aromatic (in perfumes)	10–30 grains
Osier Willow	*Salix viminalis*	Bark	Febrifuge, Tonic, Astringent	15–30 grains
Palmetto	*Sabal palmetto*	Berries	Diuretic, Tonic	10–20 grains
Pansy	*Viola tricolor*	Herb	Depurative, Laxative, Pectoral	30–60 grains
Papaya	*Carica papaya*	Juice	Vegetable Digestant	5–10 grains
Papoose Root—See **Blue Cohosh**				
Paprika—See **Cayenne Pepper**				
Paradise Grains—See **Grains of Paradise**				
Paraguay Tea—See **Maté**				
Pareira Brava	*Cissampelos pareira*	Root	Diuretic	30–60 grains
Parilla, Yellow—See **Yellow Parilla**				
Parsley	*Petroselinum sativum*	Herb	Diuretic, Febrifuge	60 grains

*For definitions of terms in "Actions and Uses" column, see pp. 178–182.
**For equivalent measures, see table of weights and measures, p. 81.

Materia Medica (continued)

PLANT NAME COMMON	LATIN	PART USED	ACTIONS AND USES*	DOSAGE**
Parsley		Root	Diuretic	30 grains
(continued)		Seeds	Diuretic, Stimulant, Emmenagogue	30 grains
Parsley Piert	*Alchemilla arvensis*	Herb	Diuretic	60 grains
Partridge Berry	*Mitchella repens*	Herb	Anti-periodic, Alterative, Diuretic	30–60 grains
Passion Flower	*Passiflora incarnata*	Herb	Diuretic, Nephritic	3–10 grains
Patchouly	*Pogostemon cablin*	Herb	Used against moths and fleas; in perfumes	

Paul's Bethony Plant—See Bugleweed
Pawpaw—See Papaya

Peach	*Prunus persica*	Leaves	Sedative, Laxative, Bitter tonic, Diuretic	30 grains

Pearl Moss—See Irish Moss

Pellitory	*Anacyclus pyrethrum*	Root	Acrid, Stimulant	2–4 grains
Pennyroyal	*Hedeoma pulegioides*	Herb	Emmenagogue, Carminative, Diaphoretic	60–120 grains

Pennywort, Indian—See Indian Pennywort

Peony	*Paeonia foemina*	Root	Antispasmodic, Tonic, Anti-epileptic	15–30 grains

*For definitions of terms in "Actions and Uses" column, see pp. 178–182.
**For equivalent measures, see table of weights and measures, p. 81.

PLANT NAME COMMON	LATIN	PART USED	ACTIONS AND USES*	DOSAGE**
		Flowers	Antispasmodic, Tonic, Anti-epileptic	60 grains
Pepper, Black	*Piper nigrum*	Fruit	Stimulant, Spice	5–20 grains
Pepper, Long—See Jaborandi				
Pepper, Red—See Cayenne Pepper				
Pepper, White—See Pepper, Black				
Peppermint	*Mentha piperita*	Leaves	Stomachic, Stimulant, Carminative, Antispasmodic	60 grains
Peruvian Balsam—See Balsam, Peru				
Peruvian Bark—See Cinchona				
Pewterwort—See Scouring Rush				
Physic, Indian—See Indian Physic				
Physic Root—See Culver's Root				
Pichi	*Fabiana imbricata*	Tops	Diuretic, Tonic, Cholagogue	
Pilewort—See Amaranth				
Pimento	*Pimenta dioica*	Fruit	Stimulant, Spice, Stomachic	10–40 grains
Pimpernel	*Pimpinella saxifraga*	Root	Expectorant, Stomachic	30 grains
Pimpernel, Red—See Red Chickweed				
Pink Root	*Spigelia marilandica*	Root	Vermifuge	60–120 grains
Pine	*Pinus* species	Needles	Expectorant; used for baths	

*For definitions of terms in "Actions and Uses" column, see pp. 178–182.
**For equivalent measures, see table of weights and measures, p. 81.

PLANT NAME COMMON	LATIN	PART USED	ACTIONS AND USES*	DOSAGE**
Pine (continued)		Buds	Expectorant, Anti-rheumatic	15–30 grains
		Gum	Used in ointments	
Pipe Plant—See Ice Plant				
Pipsissewa	*Chimaphila umbellata*	Leaves	Diuretic, Astringent, Tonic	30–90 grains
Plantain	*Plantago officinalis* and var. spp.	Herb	Pectoral, Antiseptic, Diuretic, Vulnerary	60 grains
Plantain, Branching—See Psyllium				
Plantain, Snake—See Snake Plantain				
Pleurisy Root	*Asclepias tuberosa*	Root	Expectorant, Antispasmodic, Carminative, Diuretic	20–30 grains
Plum, Wild	*Prunus vulgaris*	Bark	Expectorant, Tonic	30–60 grains
Poke	*Phytolacca americana*	Root	Alterative	1–5 grains
			Emetic	20–30 grains
		Berries	Cathartic, Alterative, Coloring	30 grains
Polecat Weed—See Skunk Cabbage				
Polygala	*Polygala amara*	Herb	Expectorant, Diuretic	30 grains

*For definitions of terms in "Actions and Uses" column, see pp. 178–182.
**For equivalent measures, see table of weights and measures, p. 81.

PLANT NAME COMMON	LATIN	PART USED	ACTIONS AND USES*	DOSAGE**
Pomegranate	*Punica granatum*	Bark of root	Anthelmintic (for tapeworm)	1–2 ounces
Pond Lily, White	*Nymphaea odorata*	Root	Astringent, Styptic, Vulnerary	30–60 grains
Poplar, Black	*Populus nigra*	Buds	Pectoral, Vulnerary	60 grains
Poplar, White	*Populus tremuloides*	Bark	Tonic, Febrifuge, Stomachic	30–60 grains
Poppy, Blue	*Papaver caeruleum*	Seeds	Edible; fed to birds	
Poppy, California	*Eschscholzia californica*	Herb	Hypnotic, Anodyne	60 grains
Poppy, Red (Corn)	*Papaver rhoeas*	Flowers	Pectoral, Emollient	15–60 grains
Prairie Pine—See Button Snakeroot				
Prickly Ash	*Zanthoxylum clava-herculis*	Bark	Tonic, Alterative, Stimulant	15 grains
		Berries	Tonic, Alterative, Stimulant	30 grains
Primrose—See Cowslip				
Prince's Feather—See Amaranth				
Prince's Pine—See Pipsissewa				
Psyllium	*Plantago psyllium*	Seeds	Laxative, Emollient	60–240 grains
Puccoon, Red—See Blood Root				
Puccoon, Yellow—See Golden Seal				

*For definitions of terms in "Actions and Uses" column, see pp. 178–182.
**For equivalent measures, see table of weights and measures, p. 81.

PLANT NAME COMMON	LATIN	PART USED	ACTIONS AND USES*	DOSAGE**
Pulsatilla—See **Meadow Anemone**				
Pumpkin	*Cucurbita pepo*	Seeds	Anthelmintic	1–2 ounces
Purging Cassia	*Cassia fistula*	Pods	Cathartic, Laxative	60–240 grains
Purshiana—See **Cascara Sagrada**				
Putcha Pat—See **Patchouly**				
Pyrethrum—See **Dalmatian Insect Powder**				
Quassia	*Simarouba excelsa*	Wood (chips)	Stomachic, Anthelmintic, Febrifuge	20–60 grains
Queen's Delight—See **Queen's Root**				
Queen of the Meadow	*Eupatorium purpureum*	Root	Diuretic, Tonic	30 grains
		Leaves	Diuretic, Astringent, Tonic	60 grains
Queen's Root	*Stillingia sylvatica*	Root	Hepatic, Depurative, Alterative	30–60 grains
Quillaya Bark—See **Soap Bark**				
Quince	*Cydonia oblonga*	Seeds	Mucilaginous (in hair setting lotion)	
Raccoon Berry—See **Mandrake**				
Ragweed	*Ambrosia artemisiifolia*	Herb	Febrifuge, Tonic	30–60 grains
Rape	*Brassica napus*	Seeds	Edible	
Raspberry	*Rubus idaeus*	Dried fruit	Diaphoretic, Febrifuge	60 grains

*For definitions of terms in "Actions and Uses" column, see pp. 178–182.
**For equivalent measures, see table of weights and measures, p. 81.

PLANT NAME COMMON	LATIN	PART USED	ACTIONS AND USES*	DOSAGE**
		Leaves	Tonic, Stimulant	30–60 grains
Rattlebush—See **Wild Indigo**				
Rattlesnake Master Root—See **Button Snakeroot**				
Rattlesnake Root—See **Black Cohosh**				
Red Chickweed	*Anagallis arvensis*	Plant	Nervine, Stimulant, Pectoral	5–15 grains
Red Clover—See **Clover, Red**				
Red Rroot	*Ceanothus americana*	Bark of root	Stimulant, Expectorant, Astringent, Sedative	30–60 grains
Red Saunders	*Pterocarpus santalinus*	Wood	Red coloring agent	
Rest Harrow	*Ononis spinosa*	Root	Tonic	30–60 grains
Rhatany	*Krameria triandra*	Root	Astringent, Tonic	15–30 grains
Rheumatism Root—See **Twin Leaf**				
Rheumatism Weed—See **Pipsissewa**				
Rhubarb	*Rheum officinale* and var. spp.	Root	Stomachic	5–10 grains
			Purgative	20–30 grains
Ribwort—See **Plantain**				
Rock Rose	*Helianthemum corymbosum*	Herb	Astringent, Tonic, Depurative	30–60 grains

---

*For definitions of terms in "Actions and Uses" column, see pp. 178–182.
**For equivalent measures, see table of weights and measures, p. 81.

PLANT NAME COMMON	LATIN	PART USED	ACTIONS AND USES*	DOSAGE**
Rocky Mountain Grape Root—See Oregon Grape Root				
Rose Hips	*Rosa villosa*	Fruit	Diuretic	30–60 grains
Rose, Red	*Rosa gallica*	Petals	Astringent	
Rose, White	*Rosa centifolia*	Petals	Aromatic	
Rosemary	*Rosmarinus officinalis*	Leaves	Stomachic, Diuretic, Aromatic, Nervine	30–60 grains
Rue	*Ruta graveolens*	Herb	Nervine, Stomachic, Vermifuge, Tonic	10–30 grains
Rupturewort	*Herniaria glabra*	Plant	Diuretic, Astringent	30–60 grains
Rush, Scouring—See Scouring Rush				
Sabadilla	*Sabadilla officinale*	Seeds	Parasiticide	
Sacred Bark—See Cascara Sagrada				
Safflower—See Saffron, American				
Saffron, American (Dyers')	*Carthamus tinctoria*	Flowers	Diuretic, Diaphoretic (in measles)	30–60 grains
Saffron, Spanish	*Crocus sativus*	Flowers	Stomachic, Antispasmodic, Stimulant, Spice	10–30 grains
Sage, Garden	*Salvia officinalis*	Leaves	Astringent, Expectorant, Spice	20–60 grains
Sage, Indian—See Boneset				

*For definitions of terms in "Actions and Uses" column, see pp. 178–182.
**For equivalent measures, see table of weights and measures, p. 81.

PLANT NAME COMMON	LATIN	PART USED	ACTIONS AND USES*	DOSAGE**
Sage, Mountain	*Artemisia frigida*	Leaves	Expectorant, Astringent, Febrifuge (in night sweats)	30–60 grains
Sage, Wild	*Salvia lyrata*	Leaves	Expectorant, Relieves inflammation	30–60 grains
Saint James Weed—See **Shepherd's Purse**				
Saint John's Bread	*Ceratonia siliqua*	Fruit	Edible, Mild laxative	
Saint John'swort	*Hypericum perforatum*	Herb	Styptic, Nervine, Pectoral	30–60 grains
Salep	*Orchis mascula* and var. spp.	Root	Demulcent, Farinaceous nutritive food	
Salt Rheum Weed—See **Balmony**				
Sampson Snakeroot—See **Gentian, Blue**				
Sandalwood, Red—See **Red Saunders**				
Sandalwood, White (Yellow)	*Santalum album*	Wood	Aromatic	
Sandarac	*Tetraclinis articulata*	Gum	Mild stimulant	
Sanicle, European	*Sanicula europaea*	Herb	Stomachic, Vulnerary, Astringent	30–60 grains
Sarsaparilla	*Smilax aristolochiifolia*	Root	Depurative, Anti-rheumatic, Alterative	30–60 grains
Sarsaparilla, Texas—See **Yellow Parilla**				

---

*For definitions of terms in "Actions and Uses" column, see pp. 178–182.
**For equivalent measures, see table of weights and measures, p. 81.

PLANT NAME COMMON	LATIN	PART USED	ACTIONS AND USES*	DOSAGE**
Sassafras	*Sassafras albidum*	Bark	Depurative, Stimulant, Diuretic, Diaphoretic	30–60 grains
		Pith	Demulcent, Ophthalmicum	30–60 grains
Savin	*Juniperus sabina*	Leaves	Diuretic, Emmenagogue, Irritant	5–10 grains
Savory, Summer	*Satureja hortensis*	Herb	Carminative, Stimulant, Spice	30–60 grains
Saw Palmetto	*Serenoa repens*	Berries	Diuretic, Tonic	10–20 grains
Saxifrage—See Pimpernel				
Scammony	*Convolvulus scammonia*	Gum resin	Cathartic	2–5 grains
Scotch Pine	*Pinus sylvestris*	Volatile oil	Anti-rheumatic (in liniments)	
		Gum	In plasters and salves	
Scouring Rush	*Equisetum arvense*	Herb	Nephritic, Astringent, Emollient	60 grains
Scrofula Plant—See Frostwort				
Scullcap	*Scutellaria laterifolia*	Herb	Tonic, Nervine, Antispasmodic	30–90 grains
Scurvy Grass	*Cochlearia officinalis*	Leaves	Antiscorbutic	30–60 grains
Sea Oak—See Sea Wrack				
Sea Onion—See Squills				

*For definitions of terms in "Actions and Uses" column, see pp. 178–182.
**For equivalent measures, see table of weights and measures, p. 81.

PLANT NAME COMMON	LATIN	PART USED	ACTIONS AND USES*	DOSAGE**
Sea Wrack	*Fucus versiculosis*	Sea plant	Alterative, Anti-fat	10–30 grains
Senega Snakeroot	*Polygala senega*	Root	Expectorant, Diuretic, Emetic	15–20 grains
Senna	*Cassia senna*	Leaves	Cathartic, Depurative	30–120 grains
		Pods	Cathartic, Depurative	30–120 grains
Serpentaria—See **Virginia Snakeroot**				
Sesame	*Sesamum indicum*	Oil	Emollient, Mucilaginous, Vulnerary; used in the arts.	
		Seeds	Used as food	
Seven Barks—See **Hydrangea**				
Shave Grass—See **Scouring Rush**				
Sheep Sorrel	*Rumex acetosa*	Leaves	Diuretic	15–30 grains
Shepherd's Purse	*Capsella bursa-pastoris*	Herb	Styptic, Astringent, Febrifuge, Diuretic	30 grains
Silkweed—See **Pleurisy Root**				
Silver Lear—See **Queen's Root**				
Silver Weed	*Potentilla anserina*	Leaves	Tonic, Astringent	30–60 grains
Simaruba	*Simaruba officinalis*	Bark	Febrifuge, Stomachic	20–60 grains
Simpler's Joy—See **Vervain**				

*For definitions of terms in "Actions and Uses" column, see pp. 178–182.
**For equivalent measures, see table of weights and measures, p. 81.

PLANT NAME COMMON	LATIN	PART USED	ACTIONS AND USES*	DOSAGE**
Skunk Cabbage	*Spathyema foetida*	Root	Expectorant, Nervine, Antispasmodic, Anti-epileptic	10–20 grains
Slippery Elm	*Ulmus fulva*	Bark	Expectorant, Diuretic, Aperient	60–120 grains
Sloe Tree	*Prunus spinosa*	Flowers	Depurative, Aperient	30–60 grains
		Berries	Astringent	30–60 grains
Smart Weed—See Water Pepper				
Snake Head—See Balmony				
Snake Lily—See Blue Flag				
Snake Plantain	*Plantago lanceolata*	Leaves	Vulnerary, Astringent	30–60 grains
Snakeroot, Black—See Black Cohosh				
Snakeroot, Button—See Button Snakeroot				
Snakeroot, Canada	*Asarum canadense*	Root	Stimulant, Carminative, Diaphoretic	15–30 grains
Snakeroot, Virginia	*Aristolochia serpentina*	Root	Febrifuge, Stimulant, Diaphoretic	15–30 grains
Soap Bark	*Quillaja saponaria*	Bark	Febrifuge, Expectorant, Saponaceous (washing delicate fabrics)	5–10 grains

*For definitions of terms in "Actions and Uses" column, see pp. 178–182.
**For equivalent measures, see table of weights and measures, p. 81.

PLANT NAME COMMON	LATIN	PART USED	ACTIONS AND USES[*]	DOSAGE[**]
Soap Wort	*Saponaria officinalis*	Herb	Saponaceous, Diaphoretic, Alterative	5–15 grains
Solomon's Seal	*Polygonatum officinale*	Root	Tonic, Astringent, Expectorant	30–60 grains
Southernwood	*Artemisia abrotanum*	Herb	Carminative, Antispasmodic	30–60 grains
Spearmint	*Mentha spicata*	Leaves	Carminative, Aromatic, Antispasmodic	60 grains
Speedwell	*Veronica officinalis*	Herb	Expectorant, Diuretic, Tonic	30–60 grains
Spicewood	*Laurus benzoin*	Bark	Aromatic, Stimulant, Febrifuge	30 grains
Spigelia—See **Pink Root**				
Spignet—See **Spikenard**				
Spikenard, American	*Aralia racemosa*	Root	Depurative, Pectoral, Stimulant, Diaphoretic, Alterative	20–30 grains
Spinach	*Spinacea oleracea*	Dried, Powdered	Rich in iron	60 grains
Spindle Tree—See **Wahoo**				
Spotted Cranesbill—See **Cranesbill**				
Spotted Knot Weed	*Polygonum persicaria*	Herb	Vulnerary, Antiseptic	30 grains

*For definitions of terms in "Actions and Uses" column, see pp. 178–182.
**For equivalent measures, see table of weights and measures, p. 81.

PLANT NAME COMMON	LATIN	PART USED	ACTIONS AND USES*	DOSAGE**
Spotted Wintergreen	*Chimaphila maculata*	Plant	Diuretic, Tonic, Alterative	30–90 grains
Spruce, Black	*Picea mariana*	Gum	Expectorant, Chewing Gum	
Spruce Bark	*Picea* spp.	Bark	Astringent	30–60 grains
Spunk—See **Larch Agaric**				
Squaw Bush— See **Cramp Bark**				
Squaw Mint—See **Pennyroyal**				
Squaw Vine—See **Partridge Berry**				
Squaw Weed—See **Life Root**				
Squills	*Urginea maritima*	Bulbs	Expectorant, Diuretic	1–2 grains
Staggerweed—See **Larkspur**				
Staphisagria—See **Staveacre**				
Star Anise	*Illicium verum*	Seeds	Stimulant, Carminative, Aromatic, Spice	15–30 grains
Star Bloom—See **Pink Root**				
Star Grass	*Hypoxis erecta*	Root	Stomachic, Tonic, Female regulator	30 grains
Starwort—See **Chickweed**				
Staveacre	*Delphinium staphisagria*	Seeds	Insecticide, Poison	
Stepmother Herb—See **Pansy**				
Stillingia—See **Queen's Root**				
Stinging Nettle	*Urtica dioica*	Herb	Diuretic, Pectoral	30–60 grains
Stingless Nettle—See **Blind Nettle**				

*For definitions of terms in "Actions and Uses" column, see pp. 178–182.
**For equivalent measures, see table of weights and measures, p. 81.

Materia Medica (continued)

PLANT NAME COMMON	LATIN	PART USED	ACTIONS AND USES*	DOSAGE**
Stoneroot—See **Collinsonia**				
Storax Balsam	*Liquidambar orientalis*	Balsam	Stimulant, Expectorant, Antiseptic in scabies	10–20 grains
Storksbill—See **Cranesbill**				
Stramonium	*Datura stramonium*	Leaves	Narcotic, Antispasmodic, Sedative, Poison	3 grains
		Seeds	Antispasmodic, Narcotic, Sedative, Bird food	3 grains
Strawberry	*Fragaria vesca*	Leaves	Diuretic, Tonic	30–60 grains
Styrax—See **Storax**				
Sumach	*Rhus glabra*	Bark	Astringent, Antiseptic	15 grains
		Berries	Astringent, Refrigerant, Diuretic	15–30 grains
Sumbul—See **Musk Root**				
Summer Savory—See **Savory, Summer**				
Sundew	*Drosera rotundifolia*	Herb	Pectoral, Rubefacient	30–60 grains
Sunflower	*Helianthus annuus*	Seeds	Bird seed	
Sunflower, Red	*Rudbeckia purpurea*	Root	Depurative	15–30 grains
Swamp Alder—See **Tag Alder**				

*For definitions of terms in "Actions and Uses" column, see pp. 178–182.
**For equivalent measures, see table of weights and measures, p. 81.

PLANT NAME COMMON	LATIN	PART USED	ACTIONS AND USES*	DOSAGE**
Swamp Cabbage—See Skunk Cabbage				
Swamp Dogwood	*Cornus sericea*	Bark	Febrifuge, Tonic, Astringent	30–60 grains
Sweet Basil—See Basil				
Sweet Birch—See Birch, Black				
Sweet Fern	*Comptonia peregrina*	Leaves	Tonic, Expectorant, Astringent	15–30 grains
Sweet Flag	*Acorus calamus*	Root	Stomachic, Carminative, Stimulant	15–30 grains
Sweet Gum—See Gum Tree				
Sweet Marjoram	*Origanum majorana*	Herb	Stimulant, Spice	30–60 grains
Sweet Wood—See Licorice				
Sweetwood Bark—See Cascarilla				
Tag Alder	*Alnus rubra*	Bark	Tonic, Astringent, Alterative	30–60 grains
Tamarack	*Larix americana*	Bark	Tonic, Laxative	15–30 grains
Tamarind	*Tamarindus indica*	Fruit pulp	Febrifuge, Mild laxative	60–240 grains
Tansy	*Tanacetum vulgare*	Herb	Emmenagogue, Vermifuge, Diaphoretic	30–60 grains
Tarragon	*Artemisia dracunculus*	Herb	Stimulant, Spice	30 grains
Tartarean Moss	*Lecanora tartarea*	Plant	Dyes red to purple	

*For definitions of terms in "Actions and Uses" column, see pp. 178–182.
**For equivalent measures, see table of weights and measures, p. 81.

| PLANT NAME | | PART | ACTIONS AND | |
COMMON	LATIN	USED	USES*	DOSAGE**
Tar Weed—See **Yerba Santa**				
Tetterwort—See **Great Celandine**				
Thimbleberry—See **Blackberry**				
Thimble Weed	*Rudbeckia laciniata*	Plant	Diuretic, Tonic, Nephritic	15–30 grains
Thistle, Blessed—See **Blessed Thistle**				
Thornapple—See **Stramonium**				
Thoroughwort—See **Boneset**				
Thousand Leaf—See **Yarrow**				
Throat Root—See **Water Avens**				
Throatwort—See **Button Snakeroot**				
Thyme, Garden	*Thymus vulgaris*	Herb	Stimulant, Spice	30–60 grains
Thyme, Wild	*Thymus serpyllum*	Herb	Stimulant, Spice	30–60 grains
Tilia—See **Linden; Basswood**				
Tobacco, English	*Nicotiana rustica*	Leaves	Expectorant, Demulcent, Tonic	60–120 grains
Tobacco, Indian—See **Lobelia**				
Tolu, Balsam—See **Balsam, Tolu**				
Tonka Bean	*Dipteryx odorata*	Fruit	Aromatic, in perfumes	
Toothache Tree—See **Prickly Ash**				
Tormentil	*Potentilla erecta*	Root	Styptic, Astringent, Tonic	30–60 grains
Tragacanth Gum	*Astragalus gummifer* and var. spp.	Gum	Mucilaginous	

*For definitions of terms in "Actions and Uses" column, see pp. 178–182.
**For equivalent measures, see table of weights and measures, p. 81.

PLANT NAME COMMON	LATIN	PART USED	ACTIONS AND USES*	DOSAGE**
Trailing Arbutus	*Epigaea repens*	Herb	Diuretic, Astringent, Tonic	60 grains
Tree Lungwort—See Lung Moss				
Trumpet Weed—See Queen of the Meadow				
Tulip Tree	*Liriodendron tulipifera*	Bark	Febrifuge, Stimulant	30–60 grains
Turkey Corn	*Dicentra canadensis*	Root	Diuretic, Tonic	10–30 grains
Turmeric	*Curcuma domestica*	Root	Stimulant, Spice	15–30 grains
Turnip, Dragon—See Indian Turnip				
Turnip, Wild—See Indian Turnip				
Turpeth Root	*Operculina turpethum*	Root	Cathartic	5–20 grains
Turtlebloom—See Balmony				
Twin Leaf	*Jeffersonia diphylla*	Root	Anti-rheumatic, Alterative, Diuretic	15–30 grains
Unicorn Root, False—See Helonias				
Unicorn Root, True	*Aletris farinosa*	Root	Stomachic, Diuretic, Female regulator, Stimulant, Aphrodisiac	15–30 grains
Unkum	*Senecio gracilis*	Herb	Emmenagogue, Diaphoretic	30–60 grains
Uva Ursi	*Arctostaphylos uva-ursi*	Leaves	Diuretic, Astringent, Tonic	20–60 grains

*For definitions of terms in "Actions and Uses" column, see pp. 178–182.
**For equivalent measures, see table of weights and measures, p. 81.

Materia Medica (continued)

PLANT NAME COMMON	LATIN	PART USED	ACTIONS AND USES*	DOSAGE**
Valerian	Valeriana officinalis	Root	Nervine, Antispasmodic, Tonic	10–15 grains
Vanilla	Vanilla planifolia	Beans	Stimulant, Flavoring	3–5 grains
Vanilla Leaf	Liatris odoratissima	Leaves	Tonic, Stimulant, Aromatic, Diaphoretic	15–20 grains
Vernal Grass, Sweet	Anthoxanthum odoratum	Plant	Aromatic, Fragrance, Perfume	15–30 grains
Veronica—See **Speedwell**				
Vervain	Verbena hastata	Herb	Antispasmodic, Expectorant, Vermifuge, Vulnerary	15 grains
Vetivert	Vetiveria zizanoides	Root	Tonic, Stimulant, In perfumes	15–30 grains
Vine Maple—See **Yellow Parilla**				
Violet	Viola odorata	Leaves	Depurative, Cathartic, Lithotropic, Discutient	30–60 grains
		Flowers	Depurative, Cathartic, Lithotropic, Discutient	30–60 grains
Virginia Snakeroot—See **Snakeroot, Virginia**				

*For definitions of terms in "Actions and Uses" column, see pp. 178–182.
**For equivalent measures, see table of weights and measures, p. 81.

PLANT NAME COMMON	LATIN	PART USED	ACTIONS AND USES*	DOSAGE**
Wafer Ash	*Ptelea trifoliata*	Bark	Tonic, Anti-periodic, Alterative, Stimulant	30–60 grains
Wahoo	*Euonymus atropurpurea*	Bark	Laxative, Diuretic, Alterative, Stimulant	8–10 grains
Wake Robin Root—See Beth Root				
Wallflower—See Bitter Root				
Wallwort—See Dwarf Elder				
Walnut, Black	*Juglans nigra*	Leaves	Depurative, Tonic	30–60 grains
		Hulls	Hair coloring	
		Bark	Astringent, Tonic	30–60 grains
Water Avens	*Geum rivale*	Root	Stomachic, Astringent, Tonic, Febrifuge	20–60 grains
Water Cress	*Nasturtium officinale*	Plant	Depurative, Antiscorbutic	30–60 grains
Water Dock	*Rumex aquaticus, R. britannica*	Root	Depurative, Alterative	30–60 grains
Water Eryngo	*Eryngium aquaticum*	Root	Diuretic, Diaphoretic	15–30 grains
Water Fennel	*Oenanthe aquatica*	Seeds	Expectorant, Carminative, Diuretic	5–10 grains

*For definitions of terms in "Actions and Uses" column, see pp. 178–182.
**For equivalent measures, see table of weights and measures, p. 81.

PLANT NAME COMMON	LATIN	PART USED	ACTIONS AND USES*	DOSAGE**
Water Hemlock—See **Water Fennel**				
Water Horehound—See **Bugleweed**				
Watermelon	_Citrullus lanatus_	Seeds	Diuretic, Mucilaginous	60–120 grains
Water Mint	_Mentha aquatica_	Herb	Stomachic, Antispasmodic, Carminative	30–60 grains
Water Pepper	_Polygonum punctatum_	Herb	Diuretic, Diaphoretic, Astringent	15–30 grains
Water Plantain	_Alisma plantago_	Leaves	Diuretic, Antilithic	30–60 grains
Water Shamrock—See **Buckbean**				
White Agaric—See **Larch Agaric**				
White Ash—See **Ash, White**				
White Bryony	_Bryonia alba_	Root	Anti-rheumatic, Drastic cathartic, Hydragogue	10–30 grains
White Nettle—See **Blind Nettle**				
White Pond Lily—See **Pond Lily, White**				
Whortleberry	_Vaccinium myrtillus_	Berry	Antiscorbutic, Astringent, Antiseptic	60–120 grains
		Leaves	Astringent, Antiseptic in Diabetes	30–60 grains
Wild Carrot	_Daucus carota_	Root	Stimulant, Diuretic, Carminative	

*For definitions of terms in "Actions and Uses" column, see pp. 178–182.
**For equivalent measures, see table of weights and measures, p. 81.

PLANT NAME COMMON	LATIN	PART USED	ACTIONS AND USES*	DOSAGE**
Wild Carrot *(continued)*		Seeds	Stimulant, Diuretic, Carminative	
Wild Cherry	*Prunus virginiana*	Bark	Expectorant, Astringent, Tonic	30–60 grains
Wild Ginger—See Snakeroot, Canada				
Wild Indigo	*Baptisia tinctoria*	Root	Stimulant, Purgative, Vulnerary	5–20 grains
Wild Sage—See Sage, Wild				
Wild Thyme—See Thyme, Wild				
Wild Turnip—See Indian Turnip				
Wild Yam	*Dioscorea villosa*	Root	Antispasmodic, Anti-bilious	30–60 grains
Willow, Black	*Salix nigra*	Bark	Anti-periodic Anti-rheumatic, Antiseptic, Astringent	15–30 grains
Willow, White	*Salix alba*	Bark	Febrifuge, Tonic, Astringent	15–30 grains
Wintergreen	*Gualtheria procumbens*	Herb	Anti-periodic, Diuretic, Alterative	60–120 grains
Witch Hazel	*Hamamelis virginiana*	Bark	Astringent, Sedative, Anti-phlogistic, Tonic	30–60 grains
Wood Betony	*Betonica officinalis*	Herb	Nervine, Cordial, Tonic	30–60 grains

*For definitions of terms in "Actions and Uses" column, see pp. 178–182.
**For equivalent measures, see table of weights and measures, p. 81.

PLANT NAME COMMON	LATIN	PART USED	ACTIONS AND USES*	DOSAGE**
Woodruff	*Galium odoratum*	Herb	Aromatic, Tonic	30–60 grains
Wormseed, American	*Chenopodium ambrosioides*	Fruit	Anthelmintic	20–40 grains
Wormseed, Levant	*Artemisia cina*	Flowers (unexpanded)	Anthelmintic	20–60 grains
Wormwood	*Artemisia absinthium*	Herb	Hepatic, Stomachic, Tonic	15–20 grains
Wormwood, Roman	*Artemisia pontica*	Herb	Astringent, Tonic	15–30 grains
Wrack, Sea—See **Sea Wrack**				
Yam, Wild—See **Wild Yam**				
Yarrow	*Achillea millefolium*	Herb	Astringent, Stomachic, Diuretic	30–60 grains
		Flowers	Astringent, Stomachic, Diuretic, Tonic	30–60 grains
Yarrow, Noble	*Achillea nobilis*	Herb	Astringent, Stomachic, Diuretic	30–60 grains
Yaw Root—See **Queen's Root**				
Yellow Dock	*Rumex crispus*	Root	Astringent, Depurative, Alterative	30–60 grains
Yellow Jessamine	*Gelsemium sempervirens*	Root	Antispasmodic, Anti-rheumatic, Febrifuge, Nervine	½–2 grains

*For definitions of terms in "Actions and Uses" column, see pp. 178–182.
**For equivalent measures, see table of weights and measures, p. 81.

Materia Medica (continued)

PLANT NAME COMMON	LATIN	PART USED	ACTIONS AND USES*	DOSAGE**
Yellow Ladies' Slipper	Cypripedium pubescens	Root	Antispasmodic, Nervine, Stimulant	10–15 grains
Yellow Moccasin Flower—See Yellow Ladies' Slipper				
Yellow Parilla	Menispermum canadense	Root	Laxative, Diuretic, Tonic	30–60 grains
Yellow Root	Xanthorrhiza apiifolia	Root	Stomachic	20–40 grains
Yerba Buena	Micromeria douglassi	Herb	Carminative, Stomachic, Febrifuge	30–60 grains
Yerba Maté—See Maté				
Yerba Rheuma	Frankinea grandifolia	Plant	Astringent, Antiseptic	10–20 grains
Yerba Santa	Eriodyctyon californica	Leaves	Expectorant	15–60 grains
Ylang-Ylang	Cananga odorata	Oil	Perfume	
Yohimbe	Corynanthe yohimbe	Bark	Aphrodisiac, Tonic	5–10 grains
Yucca	Yucca elata & var. spp.	Root	Saponaceous	
Zedoary	Curcuma zedoaria	Root	Stomachic, Stimulant, Aromatic	10–30 grains

*For definitions of terms in "Actions and Uses" column, see pp. 178–182.
**For equivalent measures, see table of weights and measures, p. 81.

8

Index of Ailments

Index of Ailments

Belching: See *Stomach Disorders*, 66–70

Biliousness: 29–30

Biting the Fingernails: 30

Blackheads: See *Impure Blood*, 50

Bladder, Inflammation of: 30

Bladder, Gravel or Stones in: See *Stones or Gravel in Kidneys or Bladder*, 70–71

Bloating: See *Stomach Disorders*, 66–70

Blood, Impure: See *Impure Blood*, 50

Blood Pressure, High: 31

Blood Pressure, Low: 31

Bloody Stools: See *Dysentery*, 40–41

Body Odor: 32

Boils: 32

Bowels, Inflammation of: See *Diarrhea*, 39–40

Breath, Bad or Foul: *See Stomach Disorders*, 66–70

Bronchitis or Bronchial Catarrh: 32

Bruises and Sprains: 32

Bunions: 33

Burns: See *Wounds*, 75

Buzzing in the Ears: See *Earache*, 41; *Blood Pressure, High*, 31

C

Canker Sores: See *Gums, Sore*, 47; *Tonsillitis*, 73; *Stomach Disorders*, 66–70

Callus: See *Corns*, 37

Carbuncles: See *Boils and Inflamed Pimples*, 32

Catarrh: See *Nasal Catarrh*, 55

Catarrh of the Bladder: See *Bladder, Inflammation or Catarrh of*, 30

Catarrh of the Bowels: See *Diarrhea*, 39–40

Catarrh of the Bronchial Tubes: See *Bronchitis*, 32

Catarrh of the Head: See *Cold or Acute Catarrh in the Head*, 35

Catarrh of the Nose: See *Nasal Catarrh*, 55

Index of Ailments

G

Gallbladder, Inflammation of: 44–45
Gallstones: See *Gallbladder, Inflammation of*, 44–45
Gas in the Stomach: See *Stomach Disorders*, 66–70; *Biliousness*, 29–30
Gastritis: See *Stomach Disorders*, 66–70
Glands, Swollen: See *Tonsillitis*, 73
Gout: 46
Gravel: See *Stones or Gravel in Kidneys or Bladder*, 70–71
Grippe: See *Cold or Acute Catarrh in the Head*, 35
Gums, Sore, Bleeding, Spongy: 47

H

Hair, Falling Out of: See *Dandruff*, 38
Hardening of the Arteries: See *Blood Pressure, High*, 31
Hay Fever: 47
Headache: 47–48
Hearing, Hardness of: See *Cold or Acute Catarrh in the Head*, 35; *Earache*, 41
Heartburn: See *Stomach Disorders*, 66–70
Hemorrhoids: 48–49
High Blood Pressure: See *Blood Pressure, High*, 31
Hives: 49
Hoarseness and Loss of Voice: 50

I

Impotence: See *Sexual Weakness*, 63
Impure Blood: 50
Indigestion: See *Stomach Disorders*, 66–70

W

Dr. Michael A. Weiner is the author of the bestselling *Earth Medicine, Earth Foods,* as well as several books on nutrition, most recently *The Art of Feeding Children Well.* A practicing nutritionist, he holds a doctorate in nutritional ethnomedicine from the University of California at Berkeley.

Mail Order Herb Suppliers

There are many local outlets for the more common herbs in every part of the country, but the following suppliers stock virtually every herb you'll need:

Nature's Herb Co.
281 Ellis Street
San Francisco, CA 94102

Pocket Herb and Apothecary
P.O. Box 183
Fairfax, CA 94930

Aphrodisia Products
45 Washington Street
Brooklyn, NY 11201

Star & Crescent Herbs
10121 R Street
Sacramento, CA 95814